COPING WITH DEMENTIA

What Every Caregiver Needs To Know

by
Rosemary L. De Cuir

Trafford
PUBLISHING

Order this book online at www.trafford.com/06-1875
or email orders@trafford.com

Most Trafford titles are also available at major online book retailers.

Note for Librarians: A cataloguing record for this book is available from Library
and Archives Canada at www.collectionscanada.ca/amicus/index-e.html

ISBN: 978-1-4251-0118-3

*We at Trafford believe that it is the responsibility of us all, as both individuals
and corporations, to make choices that are environmentally and socially sound.
You, in turn, are supporting this responsible conduct each time you purchase a
Trafford book, or make use of our publishing services. To find out how you are
helping, please visit www.trafford.com/responsiblepublishing.html*

*Our mission is to efficiently provide the world's finest, most comprehensive
book publishing service, enabling every author to experience success.
To find out how to publish your book, your way, and have it available
worldwide, visit us online at www.trafford.com/10510*

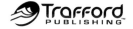

www.trafford.com

North America & international
toll-free: 1 888 232 4444 (USA & Canada)
phone: 250 383 6864 ♦ fax: 250 383 6804
email: info@trafford.com

The United Kingdom & Europe
phone: +44 (0)1865 487 395 ♦ local rate: 0845 230 9601
facsimile: +44 (0)1865 481 507 ♦ email: info.uk@trafford.com

"He shall call upon Me, and I will answer him;
I will be with him in trouble; I will deliver him and honor him"

Psalm 91:15

"When we do the best we can, we never know what miracle
is wrought in our life or in the life of another"

Helen Keller

"I know of no more encouraging fact than the unquestioned
ability of a man to elevate his life by conscious endeavor"

Henry David Thoreau

CONTENTS

DEDICATION

With deep appreciation I dedicate this book to:

My Lord, for truly apart from you I can do nothing

My parents, who live the belief that giving is a privilege, not a sacrifice.

My family, for their loyalty and support throughout the years

My friends, who "weep with those who weep and rejoice with those who rejoice"

My church family and prayer partners, who provide focus and encouragement

My colleagues, who generously share with me their expertise

My clients, past and present, who took a leap of faith by trusting my counsel

And all you kind people along the way, who kept asking if the "book was out yet"

AUTHOR'S NOTE

Once a person has clearly demonstrated that he is incapable of functioning independently in the home, it is time for the family to mobilize and work to help lessen the chances of accident, injury, or even death. It is equally important to begin to rebuild and establish a comfortable and meaningful life for your loved one. The prevailing view in today's society directly equates one's worth with what he can produce. This is similar to the nature of the sales industry – it doesn't matter how stellar past performances were – only today's results count.

Victims of dementia have no hope but to rely upon us to see them as whole persons and accept them as they are now. These are people who each have a story, a history, and a life that still has value, and it is up to us to honor their lives by treating them with as much deference as they would have received in their prime.

We each have been uniquely created, with our own blueprint. Most of us cherish our individuality and spend our lives working to leave our stamp on the world. Our American heritage and way of life especially prizes the notion of independence and self-sufficiency. Perhaps this is why dementia is feared more than many diseases, because it mercilessly strips us of our ability to think and make decisions on our own.

The subject of euthanasia has provoked torrents of controversy in our nation recently as the "usefulness" and viability of comatose patients is hotly debated. If this topic can evoke such strong reactions, I predict a fiercer storm on the horizon as more elderly people are diagnosed with a condition that produces embarrassing and undesirable behaviors. Millions are afflicted and unlike those in comas, are much more visible in society. In any case, we, as fellow citizens, must serve as proxy for those who cannot speak for themselves, and our decisions must reflect that awareness.

Dementia is a grim subject. The following pages contain much detailed and practical information, and you will have assignments to do and a great deal to organize. I have outlined the common challenges that many families face, along with suggestions and "must-knows" to help aid in achieving a successful outcome. If you are fortunate, your family will be in agreement from the onset and you can proceed relatively easily in getting the assistance you need. However, some families may face power struggles or denial and will need to find a middle ground from which to establish a common understanding in order to move things along. This book can help you identify and overcome interpersonal roadblocks that may be prohibiting you from helping your ailing loved one. It will also outline the various resources available and offer you guidance needed in order to continue to monitor your relative's care.

It is my sincere desire to help prepare you well for this journey by sharing what I have learned and offered to families facing this difficult disease. My prayer is that in these pages you will be both educated and encouraged.

Surely the noblest form of giving happens when we reach out to those who cannot possibly repay the kindness. May God bless you for your willingness to give to the needy among us.

RLD

PREFACE

In the years I spent as a community relations liaison in the retirement (and later assisted living) industry, I had the privilege of serving hundreds of families searching for appropriate housing for their parents or senior relatives. Early in my career, beginning in 1987, the term "dementia" was largely unfamiliar and had a severe connotation. Seniors showing evidence of this cognitive decline (often referred to as "senility") were deemed unsuitable for life in a retirement community and often remained at home or were sent to small board and care homes or skilled nursing facilities. Acceptance into these facilities, however, did not guarantee that the placement was appropriate or that the special needs of the individual could be met.

Support systems for families were few. There was no Internet to access for information on resources and services. Geriatric psychiatry programs and adult-day care centers were scarce. Medications were limited and often ineffective or overly powerful.

Public awareness of dementia grew largely in the 1990s due to a combination of factors including the expansion of the Alzheimer's Association, whose lobbying for research, fundraising programs and media campaigns garnered national attention. Local chapters of this powerful organization sprang up across America. Celebrity identification with the disease reinforced the fact that dementia is an indiscriminate condition that cuts across all socioeconomic lines. New information from autopsy findings, clinical trials, case studies and in-depth research by respected scientists reinforced the fact that this malady is medical in nature. MDs who previously had little exposure to this area of neuropsychiatry were able to receive additional education from colleagues specializing in the research, development and treatment of this mysterious condition.

Sadly, most Americans were made aware of the harsh reality of dementia as more and more cases were diagnosed and the disease claimed victims within their own circle of family or friends. Current estimates reveal that approximately half of those over the age of 85 are afflicted with dementia. As with alcoholism, the tentacles of this disease have reached out to so many families that an ever-growing number of people have personally been impacted by it.

The senior housing market responded to this growing phenomenon as well, first evolving from independent retirement communities to those offering assisted living services (i.e. help with bathing, dressing, medication assistance, etc.) Those diagnosed with dementia were often transferred to new "Alzheimer's wings" added to an existing community. In some cases, a facility was built servicing only those with dementia (distinguished by secured premises, specialized activities, and a daily regimen geared to stimulate and engage the resident).

Support groups, adult day and home care programs, and a variety of services also developed in the last decade as a means of offering caregivers and the afflicted needed help. Some took advantage of this, while many more families did not. It's puzzling to understand why, with an abundance of information, support and options available, did families still face such difficulty in deciding to seek assistance? Many would wait until the situation was at crisis point and as a result, hasty decisions were made often with poor or disastrous results. This reluctance to move ahead with a comprehensive plan of action still exists with many families today.

In my job I needed to audit every file and analyze why the staff of a care facility was unable to convince the family that the time had come to make a decision to move a parent into the dementia program (or merely arrange for *some* kind of short-term help). On the surface it seemed obvious to assume that families would jump at the chance to receive what the average observer would deem a lifeline. After all, these people were *seeking out information* because something at home wasn't working anymore. "They come to us desperate, I spend all this time with them, and then they do nothing about it" was a common lament our sales staff would voice. While some families were proactive, many more delayed in getting the help they needed, despite the seriousness of the situation at home. Our team would, on average, spend 2-6 months working with a family, building relationships, touring and re-touring, talking on the phone, and working to establish trust.

With the exception of the few families who had opted to move to a competitive facility, most in the "pending" file that I reviewed had made *no decision* according to follow-up made over the next six months. I found this intriguing, considering that most had stated in the initial interview notes that they were inquiring because the situation had reached a desperate point. Frustrated marketing directors that I trained complained to me that the family was procrastinating, in denial, struggling to convince a sibling, overwhelmed with guilt or just too afraid to act. "It's so obvious – why can't they see they need help?" was a frequent refrain I'd hear from staff.

I realized that it was futile to try to hammer home what we felt was common sense, as our clients were frequently intelligent, sensible people. Most of them had enough pamphlets, prices and information – they just didn't know what to do with it because the decision dealt mainly with intangibles (feelings, values) – and these weren't being addressed. These clients weren't buying a refrigerator; they were making a lifestyle change that had huge stakes attached. Instead of expecting them to trust us, we needed to learn to help them first trust themselves, and they could only do this if we helped them explore the reasons behind their reticence.

I knew that we would need to help families examine their emotional concerns and identify barriers that were obviously overriding the pressing practical needs and even good common sense of an otherwise sensible family. My goal, then, was to find a way to help families give themselves permission to admit that they were stuck and needed help dealing with an unfamiliar and frightening disease. These sons, daughters, spouses, friends and caregivers were good people who were genuinely concerned about the worsening state of a loved one, but were stalled and unable to move. I felt sympathy for these individuals and sought to reassure them that they were not, (as many of them believed) "bad kids." Bad kids, I reminded my clients, never lost a moment's sleep over the welfare of their relative. Bad kids didn't find themselves emotionally and physically spent from hours of unselfish care given. Bad kids didn't care, period.

It took some work and a lot of reinforcement to help families overcome their self-doubt and learn to pinpoint the source of their fears, but it was exciting to watch these "good kids" regain their equilibrium and develop better coping skills in order to best help their afflicted loved one. The only prerequisite for success was the willingness to try and the resolution to stick with it. In the following pages we will look at the most common reasons behind failure to act and possible origins for this behavior. I have also provided suggestions in remedying these problems – drawing from counsel that has proven to be helpful with many families that I have worked with over the years.

While the sources of dementia remain mysterious, equally perplexing are the complex feelings and responses of those dealing with the disease. Learning to push through fears and act despite the discomfort is the beginning of liberation for these families. I counsel families to put their feelings on "auto-pilot" and have enough faith in themselves to trust their decisions, but that is only the first step. Caregivers **must** also be informed and aware of the barriers they may encounter as they carry out their plan of action. These will be highlighted in the following chapters with suggestions on how to overcome them.

Once families make a concrete decision, they now need to begin to let go as they transition from the role of ***primary caregiver*** to ***advocate.*** Families can do this if they do two things – 1) **arm themselves with information** and have a clear understanding of how to proceed in enlisting the aid of professionals, screening facilities, and monitoring the care of their loved one, and 2) **accept that their role, while altered, remains equally important and will continue.** This goes a long way in eliminating misguided guilty feelings that one has "abandoned" his loved one.

In this book I have endeavored to help families in both identifying removing roadblocks (internal or external) and also to learn how to put an informed, effective plan of action in place.

This book is not clinical or medical in nature. It is meant to be a traveling companion, a guidebook. It is a compilation of information gleaned from years of serving families from all walks of life. Despite the diversity of our personalities and circumstances, we all struggle with the same self-doubts, fears, and weaknesses. For caregivers fighting the ravages of dementia, the problems seem magnified many times over. In these pages I have shared the same words of affirmation that I have offered my clients through the years with some straightforward advice as well.

In deference to the reader, I have opted not to identify the individual as a "patient" nor use the term "demented" (some physicians prefer "brain-injured"). As most cases of dementia are diagnosed in older adults, I have used the terms "senior," and "parent" frequently, interchanged with "loved one" and "afflicted individual." I have also alternated the use of the pronouns *his* and *her* as both genders are claimed by the disease. Since the majority of caregivers reading this book are related to their charges, familial terms are used often.

May each page encourage and enlighten you on your journey.

1

UNDERSTANDING DEMENTIA

WHAT IT IS
Dementia is the medical term for a group of symptoms that indicate a significant decline in cognitive functioning and intellectual ability. The decline is marked enough to interfere with an individual's ability in several areas such as recall, judgment, memory, and daily functioning of various sorts.

There are many types of dementia, with Alzheimer's disease as the most recognizable. Some types of dementia are short-lived; for instance, those brought on by reactions to anesthesia are often temporary, while others signify the beginning of an inescapable life-long decline. Medications are often prescribed for those individuals diagnosed in the early stages of the disease. While there is no known cure at this time, some drugs have been shown to slow the progression of the dementia and/or stabilize anxious behaviors.

ORIGINS OF DEMENTIA

Dementia, which results from loss of or damage to neurons in the brain, takes many forms and is caused by many diseases or conditions, including:

- Metabolic disorders
- Structural problems in the brain (tumors, head traumas)
- Infections (AIDS, TB, syphilis)
- Degenerative diseases – Alzheimer's, Huntington's Disease, Parkinson's Disease
- Lewy-body
- Vascular (stroke, oxygen deprivation, multi-infarct)
- Psychiatric disorders (depression)
- Alcoholism
- Multiple Sclerosis, Down Syndrome
- Exposure to toxins (heavy metals, etc.)

Approximately half of those over the age of eighty-five are diagnosed with Alzheimer's disease each year. Recent estimates produced by the Alzheimer's Association indicate that approximately five million Americans suffer from this disease. The number of Americans afflicted with Alzheimer's disease has doubled in the last two years and is still growing. Average survival time depends upon various factors including patient's overall health, age, and stage of development at the time of diagnosis.

It is important to note that dementia is not the same as normal, "age-associated" memory loss (i.e., losing keys, etc.) This is a physiological impairment that can be measured in various ways and significantly disturbs the ability of one to function independently in the activities of daily living (a term you will become quite familiar with).

THREE STAGES OF DEMENTIA

In defining the progression of dementia, it is generally categorized by three stages – **early (mild)**, **middle (moderate)** and **late (severe).** These stages are distinguished by the following characteristics:

EARLY (MILD) STAGE
- Still functional, some confusion
- Increased difficulty in performing tasks
- Aware of decline in condition, fairly adept at hiding it; has "clear" days
- Can still care somewhat for self
- Requires minimal supervision (may not prepare balanced meals, skips medications, forgets to turn stove off)
- Physical condition generally good; however, hygiene may begin to be neglected
- Still may initiate conversation

MIDDLE (MODERATE) STAGE
- Confusion apparent
- Supervision needed
- Needs considerable direction/assistance
- Loss of control of bowel and bladder
- Aware of confusion but can't hide it
- Ability to communicate limited; can't express thoughts easily

LATE (SEVERE) STAGE
- Severe confusion
- Loss of all functional skills
- Caregiver meets all needs
- Ability to eat, talk, move about and recall are lost
- Unaware of condition

With Alzheimer's disease, behaviors and conditions will vary depending upon which lobes of the brain are affected. Simply put, damage to a certain lobe will impact functioning that is unique to that part of the brain. The relationship of specific functions to the respective brain lobes are categorized as follows:

Frontal lobe	memory, speaking, imagination, attention, rational thinking, judgment, cognition (inability to learn), personality
Hippocampus	skilled movements
Parietal lobe	sensory perception (pain, touch, temperature, pressure)
Temporal lobe	language, hearing, smell
Occipital lobe	visual association, depth and distance perception
Cerabellum	equilibrium
Medulla oblongota	breathing, heart rate, blood pressure

COMMONLY USED TERMS YOU MAY ENCOUNTER*

ACUITY – keenness of ability. (Term used in dementia care to describe level of functioning).

ADL's – Acronym for "activities of daily living" such as bathing, eating, dressing and toileting.

ADVANCE NOMINATION – Designates someone to serve as an individual's conservator if the court deems it necessary

ADVANCED HEALTHCARE DIRECTIVE – Authorizes a loved one or friend to make medical decisions for the designee.

AGNOSIA – Loss of ability to recognize familiar objects or stimuli

APHASIA – Loss of ability to use or comprehend words.

APRAXIA – Loss of ability to execute complicated acts or movements without the impairment of muscles or senses.

ARICEPT – (Donepezil HCI) Medication prescribed to slow progression of symptoms of the disease in mild to moderate stage patients, typically.

CONTINENCE – Ability to control bowel and bladder function.

CUSTODIAL CARE – Assistance with ADL's (not requiring a licensed nurse or therapist).

DURABLE POWER OF ATTORNEY – Person designated by court appointment to manage finances of individual deemed incapacitated.

ELDER ABUSE – Defined either by physical abuse, neglect, financial abuse, abandonment, isolation, abduction, or other treatment with resulting physical harm or pain or mental suffering; the deprivation of a care custodian of goods or services that are necessary to avoid physical harm or mental suffering.

GAIT – Manner of walking, usually refers to stability and balance of an impaired person.

GERIATRIC PSYCHIATRY – Treatment of cognitive and psychiatric disorders in geriatric population. (Some hospitals have designated a section of the neuro- psychiatric unit for inpatient evaluation and treatment of patients afflicted with dementia).

HIPAA – Health Insurance Portability and Accountability Act, designed in part to strengthen the laws regarding privacy of medical information.

MEDICARE – Federal health program that covers largely hospital and doctor bills. Medicare may also cover nursing home care if patient requires skilled care, and will only pay for the first 100 days of the patient's stay.

NAMENDA (Memantine HCI) – Medication prescribed to slow progression of dementia symptoms in moderate to severe stages of the disease

PSYCHOTROPIC – Affecting mental activity, behavior, perception; commonly refers to mood-altering drug prescribed to calm agitated individuals

RE-DIRECTION – Technique used to distract and re-focus agitated individual

REVOCABLE (LIVING) TRUST – Allows management of assets for an individual before and after his death outside of court jurisdiction, thus avoiding probate.

Familiarizing yourself with these and other terms will help you as you begin to network with service and medical professionals and providers.

Let's next look at the warning signs that can alert one to the possibility that dementia may be present in your loved one.

*Credit – California Medical Association, American Bar Association.

2

WARNING SIGNS

WHEN A FAMILY MEMBER suspects a loved one to be suffering from dementia, he needs to find out if his fears are warranted – especially if his relative lives alone. As mentioned earlier, dementia is not benign forgetfulness, but rather a marked decline in cognitive functioning, usually characterized in the following ways:

- Difficulty in discussing abstract ideas (thoughts, principles, opinions)
- Uncharacteristic and irregular emotional outbursts
- Lack of attention paid to details (mail left out for days, bills piling up or thrown out)
- Decline in self-care (forgets to eat, poor hygiene, missed appointments)
- Erratic behavior, hoarding, hiding of valuables
- Irrational fears, paranoia or delusional behavior
- Imagined insults, conversations and snubs
- Home maintenance poor, house or yard unkempt
- Withdrawal from activities previously enjoyed

- Inability to perform tasks to completion (cooking, bill-paying, operating a car,
- reading a newspaper article, putting an outfit together)
- Rituals no longer observed (skipping church, medications missed, doesn't observe holidays)

You may also observe that the car has not been used in some time, or perhaps there is evidence of new dents and damage to the vehicle. Another red flag would be the indication that your parent seems unaware of the changing of the seasons (doesn't pull out summer clothes from storage, prepare the house for cooler weather, etc.)

WHAT YOU CAN DO:

Ask any neighbors familiar with your parent to share what they know. You will want to document any incidences that they have observed. Quote them and record dates and times.

Arrive unannounced at your parent's home. Vary your visiting times (your parent may be okay in the day but really struggles after sunset).

Ask yourself if you feel comfortable going away on a long vacation and not contacting your parent. Be honest. Do you truly believe he could manage unassisted, as he did in your younger years? What if there were a natural disaster or emergency? Would your parent have the presence of mind to know what to do?

Beware of new friends, household help, romantic relationships, or renters. Confused seniors are particularly vulnerable to being swindled, as they are so easily befriended. I have worked with many families who saw their parents' entire life savings, home, and other holdings lost to charlatans who wormed their way into a position of power. Particularly vulnerable are the lonely seniors who have no children nearby. Get on a plane or have a trusted relative, neighbor or friend go visit your parent immediately. If a stranger answers the phone, ask to speak with your parent and do not be put off with the excuse that "he is napping" or in the tub. (This is a common ploy used to deter phone conversations, especially if the senior is having a "hazy" day). Get your parent on the phone. Honest people will understand that you need to protect your loved one.

Call the telephone company and arrange to have unidentified calls blocked. You don't want your parent solicited or put in the position to give out confidential information.

Check the mail. You need to find out if your parent has credit card statements that reflect a balance. All credit cards should be destroyed if your parent is unable to use them properly. Take the necessary steps to start the process. Find a copy of the telephone and utility bills and check for any unusual or excessive charges. Report anything suspicious.

If you have reason to believe that your parent's bank accounts are accessible to an outsider, **immediately notify** the bank and get those accounts closed.

Arrange to spend a few days with your parent. Engage him in conversations and try to let him do most of the talking. Have breakfast together and try to discuss a newsworthy headline. See how well he can follow the train of thought. Pay attention to sleep patterns and watch to see if regular square meals are prepared or skipped. Observe grooming regimens – have they changed? Watch to see if he is comfortable answering the telephone. Hand him the remote control to the television and see how adept he is in choosing a program. Watch a simple game show together and see if he is able to comprehend.

By now you should have an accurate assessment of your parent's capabilities. If your loved one has largely failed to prove that he is able to live safely and comfortably on his own, you must step in and play the most unnatural role there is. You must respectfully parent your parent.

3

EFFECTIVE COMMUNICATION

OFTEN IN MY WORK I would hear the lament, " I try to be sensitive when I talk to my mom, but I just seem to upset her more and we end up fighting." Why does this happen? Because the daughter, while meaning well, was using the wrong set of communication skills in trying to reach her confused parent.

Learning to communicate with one afflicted with dementia is a process. For most people, this is a skill that will need to be acquired, and developing this is a new and frustrating experience. However, if one sticks with it, he will enjoy a more calm, controlled dialogue with his loved one.

Adult children commonly complain that sometimes they can't understand why they have to change the way in which they have always spoken to their parent. They are sincere in their insistence that they are logical and respectful in their interaction.

What families need to remember is that in terms of dialogue, the playing field is no longer even. There is no longer a balanced exchange of ideas and thoughts. The parent suffers a serious impairment and must be seen as not capable of rational thought in terms of problem solving and identifying feelings. *You must acquire the skill of compassionate communication.*

COMMUNICATION TIPS:
- Remember that **logic does not** work.
- Give **brief**, one-sentence explanations.
- **Repeat** yourself.
- **Agree** with made-up stories.
- **Hear** the person out.
- Remind yourself that, by virtue of the disease, the person is **always right**. Change **your** mindset.
- **Speak simply**. Use words he understands.
- **Allow time** for response.
- Respond to the person's **feelings**, not her words.
- Do not contradict or argue, **no matter what**.
- **Do not reason** with the person.
- If you are accused of something, quietly **apologize** and change subject.
- When agitation is apparent, **acknowledge it and re-direct it** (read on for suggestions on how to accomplish this).

You need to think of your parent in a new light. You must see him with limited reasoning powers, similar to those of a young child. You wouldn't talk to your first-grader in the same way that you would speak to your best friend, would you?

In a caring manner free of condescension, you will need to guide conversations, de-personalizing them and controlling the direction of the discourse in order to achieve the right results. This requires some work.

Remind yourself that being right is not the goal – *getting the right result is.* And the right result is a calm exchange that communicates not information, but love.

WHY ARGUING DOESN'T WORK

In ordinary exchanges between people, for instance, if there were a misunderstanding on one's part, we would attempt to reason with the person to convince him logically that he was mistaken. With a person with dementia the reasoning is too abstract for the person to comprehend. Instead of being mollified, he interprets your response as an argument, a denial. You will not comfort the person by trying to reason with him – in fact, you will only make him angrier.

It takes some thinking in order to control responses with anyone, particularly someone with whom you have a long history and who now is battling dementia. However, if you want to save yourself a lot of fruitless arguments, you will want to make the effort to learn how to guide the direction of a conversation without it escalating into a war of words.

Think of this in terms of learning to excel in any disciplined game. Most of us don't grab a baseball bat and expect to hit home runs! Training, preparation and proper protective gear are necessary to aid the player. You are no different. The family that thinks they can just continue to correct mother's flubs will only succeed in starting a frustrating verbal free-for-all.

Remind yourself every time you need to interact with your parent that you need to "suit up" and you'll put yourself in the correct frame of mind for a successful exchange with that person.

Example of a well-meaning conversation headed for disaster:

Child – "Uh, mom, I was wondering if you noticed that lately you've been forgetting to take your diabetes medication."
Parent – "No, I didn't."
Child – "Yes, I saw an extra pill on the sink."
Parent – "Don't bother me."
Child – "It's just that I know those pills are important."
Parent – "I know what I'm doing."
Child – "I'm sorry, Mother."

Strike one. Two more chances at bat.

Child – "Mom, I bought this little pill holder at the store. You can separate your pills by the day."
Parent – "I don't need that."
Child – "I don't mean to nag you, but I'm worried about your skipping medications."
Parent – "I'm fine."
Child – "I know you're very capable, but I think...."
Parent – "I don't want to talk anymore."
Child – "Fine!"

Strike two. Have you noticed that the stakes are higher, the problem remains, and the irritation level on both sides is growing? Read on:

Child – "Mom, I know you don't want to hear it, but I'm tired of coming over and seeing that you've skipped your pill!"
Parent – "I did not!"
Child – "Yes, you did! Can't you see the extra one? Do you want to end up in the hospital?"
Parent – "Stay out of it!"
Child – "We have to talk about it! It's not working this way!"
Parent – "Leave me alone!"
Child – "I can't leave you alone! You can't take care of yourself!"
Parent – "Your father won't like this!"
Child – "Daddy's dead! Don't you remember?"
Parent – "You're lying!"

Strike three. As far as both players are concerned, game over. Not only has the adult child gotten nowhere in her desire to make sure mom takes her pills, but she has caused great aggravation by attempting to reason with her confused parent. The daughter needed to learn successful techniques in conveying her concern to mom in such a way that mom would not react with anger, bewilderment, or shame.

As you are "suiting up" for a conversation with your loved one, remind yourself of the following:

- I am not here to win a debate.
- I need most of all to convey my love for her.
- The subject is not the issue.
- I need to comfort, not confront.
- Reasoning and logic are not going to work – period.
- I will not convince her or change her mind. I don't need to, anyway.
- I will only make it worse if I insist on pressing my point.
- She is not able to comprehend my arguments. All she hears is a soft, kind voice or a frustrated, bossy one.
- She interprets tone and body language.

Some children will need to resist the urge to impress their parent, especially if they have a history of pleasing difficult mothers and fathers. Check your feelings at the door and deal with them later. For now, you've got survive a conversation without losing your temper or equilibrium.

HOW DEMENTIA FILTERS MESSAGES

Remember that what your parent is saying is not necessarily what she *wants* to communicate (particularly as the disease progresses). We are used to taking the literal word to represent one's position, but this is largely untrue when dealing with a dementia victim. The impaired person does not recognize language as a medium in which to express thoughts. He uses language to express **feelings**, and feelings are what the listener must focus on. A confused individual is drawing conclusions from the speaker's tone of voice, inflection and expression. Your response is interpreted as friendly or hostile, plain and simple. The **subject** of the discussion is of little actual importance.

I attended a lecture once where the guest speaker tried an

experiment on all of us. The point of this game was to bring to life the challenges that a confused person faces in trying to process information. The speaker had us put cotton balls between each finger before donning plastic gloves, place more cotton in our ears and tie a piece of plastic wrap securely over our eyes. Next, we were told to hold a pencil in the hand we normally do not write with, and we were given a strip of notepaper.

The speaker then turned up a radio that was on the center table and began to speak at a fairly rapid clip. She reeled off a list of suggestions that we were supposed to jot down – i.e., buy milk at the store, pick up dry cleaning, etc. As I struggled to keep up, I could feel different emotions swirling around in me. After the timer went off, the speaker asked us to describe our feelings during the test. Adjectives like "frustrated," "clumsy" and "inept" were used by most of the group.

"This is how persons with dementia receive messages," our speaker said. "They are filtered in a variety of ways and it gets worse with the disease."

I never forgot that lesson or the insight that it gave into the tiny world of dementia. It made me realize that I would need to do my best to reach its victims, rather than insist that they try to visit my comfortable sphere.

LEARN TO LIVE IN THE MOMENT

Remember that as time goes on, the impaired person lives increasingly "in the moment." His perception of time becomes increasingly blurred and skewed (which is why it is relatively easy for most to adapt rather quickly to change of environment, as long as routines remain the same). It is important to keep this in mind when engaging in conversation. Unless the senior is reminiscing with you about a happy past event, keep the dialogue brief and in the here and now.

The attention span of a person with dementia grows increasingly short, which is likely one reason it is usually simple to redirect an agitated individual. The challenge, however, is that the person will frequently need to be amused in a variety of ways, as she often will tire quickly of an activity. Her ability to concentrate on any given thing is compromised.

HANDLING DELUSIONAL BEHAVIOR

Typically, as the disease claims more of the person's thought processes, you may encounter delusional behavior in some cases. The person may become obsessed with the notion that he is being robbed or abused. He can become very insistent that someone is "after" him. A normally complacent individual can become easily irritated or even paranoid when he reaches this stage. Typical comments can include:

"I've been robbed again and no one is doing anything about it."
"They haven't given me a bath in three days."
"He's trying to poison me."
"I know what's going on around here – you can't fool me!"
"She's in the room, hiding from you."

WHEN BEING SENSIBLE DOESN'T MAKE SENSE

Your first normal reaction to comments like the above stated ones is to refute and correct. WRONG! You'll only encourage her fears by doing that. While everything you say may be factually true, it is meaningless in that the individual cannot comprehend its meaning.

Let's look at typical responses and compare them to the interpretations that the confused person attaches to the statements. Count on the fact that his perception of what you are trying to articulate is markedly different from your own viewpoint.

YOUR STATEMENT:	HE "HEARS":	HE "SEES"
"You live on the second floor of a secured building No one could possibly get in to rob you.".	"That's ridiculous."	Disbelief
"I know for a fact that the staff has bathed you every day."	"You are lying"	Denial
"That man is a very good employee. You'd hurt his feelings if he heard you say he was trying to poison you."	"I believe him, not you"	Disloyalty
"Nothing's going on. We all want what's best for you."	"Be quiet"	Disdain
"What an imagination you have!"	"How silly of you"	Disgust

The facts that you stated are too hazy to be sorted through, so they are discarded. What is taken into consideration is your amused smile, annoyed sigh, or dismissive attitude. <u>That</u> is understood, and it infuriates the person wildly.

CORRECT RESPONSES

**"How scary to be robbed! Let's go tell the policeman."
(Acknowledge, re-direct)**

**"That's awful! Let's draw a nice warm bath right now"
(Acknowledge, re-direct)**

**"We'll have that man arrested. You'll be safe."
(Acknowledge, comfort)**

"I know how smart you are. Let's report the troublemakers." (Acknowledge, re-direct)

"Let's go tell security about the lady in your room. They'll take her away." (Acknowledge, comfort)

In one of the facilities that I worked in, I used a police officer's cap purchased from a costume shop. If an agitated resident complained about a break-in or a conspiracy, I asked our capable receptionist to fill out a "police report" and meet with the resident. Within a few moments a friendly member of our staff would easily redirect the person to an activity or a meal.

We also found that our residents who complained about the management of the building were placated when we asked them to "run" a staff meeting, or handed them a resignation form, or gave them other opportunities in which to be heard. These residents were quickly mollified and were on to their next adventure shortly thereafter. These tactics took only a few moments to carry out and de-escalated tensions easily, and they also won the gratitude of the families.

4

LOVE ON THE ROCKS

(When Dementia Affects Relationships)

"I feel like a five year old when I'm with my mother. I know my family is disgusted – I'm disgusted with myself. Every time I resolve to be firm, Mother cries or tells me she knows she's a burden. I shut up because I feel so guilty."

I REMEMBER THIS CONVERSATION clearly. The speaker had contacted me and set an appointment to discuss having her mother move to our retirement community. "Mrs. B" came to my office accompanied by her husband, who sat defiantly silent for the first forty minutes of the interview. In this period of time, he barely made eye contact with his wife and his body language communicated great disdain. Meanwhile, the woman carried on in despair about her mother, who had come to her daughter's home for a short visit and ended up staying for seven years! Now dementia had set in and the situation was much worse. The wife was working outside the home, exhausted with keeping up with mom's ever-growing confusion, and annoyed at herself for her inability in handling a very critical, demanding parent. "Mom calls me at work seven to eight times a day. I'm worried I'll lose my job, which would help in a way, but then I'd be at home all the time with her and that would make me crazy," she declared.

To make matters worse, Mrs. B's teenage children seemed unsympathetic and disinterested in helping out much, and increasingly resentful that their mom's attention was focused mainly on their grandmother. Grandma's inconsistent behavior was sometimes downright bizarre and embarrassing when the family ate out at a restaurant or went to church together.

Most distressing to Mrs. B was the change in her husband, whose normally mild-mannered temperament was becoming peppered with angry outbursts and increasingly distant behavior. Mrs. B's misery was compounded by her own anger at herself, and her frustration with a situation described as "spiraling downward."

This woman was on thin ice. Her ability to care for her mother was dwindling, as she felt unable to continue under the weight of many responsibilities with a career and family life. Her confidence was shaky. The love and support of her husband and children, which had helped sustain her over the years, had been severely stretched and was breaking under the strain of caring for her mother. Waves of anger, fatigue and resentment were threatening to engulf the entire family.

STRAIGHT TALK FOR THE CAREGIVER

Married caregivers are all too aware (and sometimes resentful) of the fact that their spouses cannot empathize with their burden. Parent/child relationships are unique and compounded by all the complex dynamics, issues and years of history that surround them. Dementia complicates the relationship significantly and the caregiver feels more singled out than ever, despite her partner's best efforts to understand. This almost gives the caregiver permission to withdraw from the relationship.

However, this does not mean that spouses can't offer strength and assistance during this trying time. Caregivers who feel exiled in this lonely dilemma often act out this abandoned feeling to the point that they feel unreachable. **The more distant they feel, the more they act on that feeling**. They push away those who wish to help them but who are unsure of how to do it. Tensions arise, tempers fly and each side retreats to a corner. The caregiver continues in her duties, angrier and more depressed than ever. The dementia hasn't claimed her mind, just her way of life and her ability to relate to her loved ones.

Too many caregivers make the mistake of feeling entitled to set aside their responsibilities to their spouses and families, justifying this by claiming that they "only have so much to give." They view the demands of the spouse or children as unreasonable and are sometimes bitter that anything is expected of them. "Don't they understand what I have to deal with all day with Mother?" is an oft-said phrase. This attitude can all but finish off relationships that could have offered the stressed caregiver strength and support.

When I have explained this to caregivers, I would be met sometimes with annoyance. The caregiver would feel that it was unrealistic to ask *one more thing* of him in addition to their already heavy responsibilities. "Why are you siding with my husband?" was the reaction many gave me.

This was the crux of the matter, and this attitude was proof of the caregiver's misreading of the situation. *There should be no sides in this*. The caregiver must stop seeing herself as a solo force in the care of her loved one and begin to reclaim her life. The first step is to vow to honor that life by protecting it. Caregivers have an obligation to protect themselves, first and foremost, from burnout. They owe it to themselves to take good care of their physical, mental, emotional and spiritual needs. A tired, angry care manager is of no use to anyone. Dementia victims need a healthy, calm advocate.

Spouses also need well-adjusted, balanced mates.

SUREFIRE WAYS TO DO DAMAGE TO A MARRIAGE:
- *Accuse your spouse* on a regular basis of not caring. Conveniently forget that he is still a contributing part of the family.
- *Bottle up your emotions.* Share them only when you blow up in anger.
- *Misdirect your rage* at the disease toward your spouse. Spread a little misery around.
- *Be emotionally unavailable* for your spouse's needs, concerns and problems.
- *Let your physical appearance and health run down.* Life's a mess – so why not look the part?
- *Devote every bit of energy* towards your parent. Skip your children's activities, family trips, and quiet time. Let go of your interests and hobbies. Who has time to be well rounded?
- *Insist on playing the martyr.* Refuse to allow help from professionals, friends and outsiders. Do everything, drive everywhere, and handle all problems alone. Tell yourself that no one cares as much as you, and then complain how no one lifts a finger to help. Control every little detail and then be angry that your life feels out of control.
- *Think of this as your problem alone*, rather than as a family challenge.

Got the picture? Good! Of course you don't want to live this way, because you are reading this book in order to learn more about how to attack this disease. Read on and learn how to do this with the love and support of your family. We'll start by identifying the source of some relational problems and look at ways to establish patterns that re-connect partners who experience problems similar to Mr. and Mrs. B's.

WHY RELATIONSHIPS BREAK DOWN

The couples whom I've interviewed who were facing similar struggles in their relationship had several similarities:

- **They had ceased** to make their marriage top priority in their lives.
- **They had allowed** outside influences to drive a wedge in their relationship.
- **They failed to set** and enforce healthy practices and boundaries designed to protect themselves, their relationship and their family life.
- **They allowed** their daily responsibilities to overshadow their lives to the point that they lost sight of their long-term goals and plans.
- **They let** circumstances control their lives rather than the other way around.
- **They labored** under a strong sense of guilt, which overrode any other emotion or conviction.

A WORD ON GUILT

The most common phrase I would hear when working with couples was "I feel so guilty."

While some adult children have legitimate reason to make amends for misdeeds they committed against their parents, the vast majority I have worked with have a misguided sense of guilt, brought on not by *actions* but *feelings*. People who suffer from misplaced guilt open themselves up to all sorts of problems if they don't reassess their guilty feelings and properly address them.

Webster defines guilt in two ways:

- the fact of having committed a breach of conduct

or

- feelings of culpability especially for imagined offenses or from a sense of inadequacy (I call it "inappropriate guilt")

Most caregivers fall into the latter category. They are not truly guilty of misdeeds against their ailing parent. They, for a variety of reasons, simply feel that they are poorly suited to offer adequate care to the ill person. These feelings of inadequacy are so powerful that they cloud otherwise sound judgments, and the person stubbornly forges ahead – alone.

These reactions, while loving and legitimate, shape the coping patterns of caregivers, and ironically, can cause harm to the very family unit that is so cherished if the feelings alone are allowed to reign.

Instead of urging the conflicted caregivers to forget their feelings (which is impossible), I learned a better way to help them move past these very strong convictions.

The key is to remember that actions shape feelings and to start acting out with the expectation that positive feelings will follow.

TURN IT AROUND NOW

As mentioned earlier, when depressed caregivers retreat into the singular world of "self -service" they do so because they feel isolated. Their actions reinforce these feelings, which become so strong that they override the protestations of loved ones. Initial misgivings that caregivers have about this unnatural situation are rationalized away as "unloving" or "selfish." The cycle continues, until you have a scenario such as the one Mr. and Mrs. B. were facing.

BRIDGING A GAP

It took a bit of work to draw Mr. B out, which was to be expected as he felt his opinion mattered little (since his wife wasn't taking his advice). I sought to defuse his anger by first commending him for coming in to meet me, which I felt was a show of support for his wife. I asked Mr. B. to share his thoughts and opinions about the best course of action in which to help his mother-in-law (and preserve his family).

Several times Mrs. B. interrupted and I needed to politely ask her to hold her comments until we heard her husband out. At this point, Mr. B. began to open up. He sensed that I respected his position and began to freely share about the burden he felt he had carried, along with his anger at his wife for what he felt was buckling under "Mother's" pressure.

Mr. B. wasn't a bad man; in fact, he acknowledged his love for his mother-in-law and his sorrow over her condition. He was, however, straightforward in stating that he felt the family's life had been consumed by her situation and that it was out of control. He also confessed that he "didn't get" the dementia and was disturbed by the erratic behaviors that he witnessed nearly every day.

I asked Mr. B. if I might speak privately to his wife and he stepped outside. Mrs. B. immediately asked what I thought. I asked her if she wanted to stay married, and she nodded. I told her that the current arrangement was alienating her strongest advocates, and that her mother's disease was claiming more that one victim. Mrs. B. owed it to her marriage, her children and to herself to preserve these relationships and protect them at all costs. Ruining her marriage and alienating her children was not going to decrease her level of stress or help her desperately needy parent. What's more, she had shown her family disrespect by giving them the message that their needs were not a priority to her. Her actions communicated to her husband and children that she did not *trust* her family, thus further alienating them.

ENCOURAGEMENT FOR THE CAREGIVER

During this difficult time, it is important to stay positive and have clarity of thought. If you need to re-train your thoughts, replace the self-defeating ones with helpful truths. Refuse to listen to negative, helpless self-recriminations.

You can start by looking at your spouse in a new light – by imagining how you would cope if the situation were reversed and you were watching your partner struggle with a parent. Remind yourself that:

- Spouses **want to be** the best source of support for their partners.
- Your spouse **feels sympathy** for what you are enduring.
- Your spouse is **feeling left out** of the decision-making process, and as a result feels helpless to aid you. This is especially hard on men, who are "fixers" by nature.
- Your spouse **may be alarmed** that you are sinking under this burden and will do damage to your health, marriage and way of life.
- Your spouse **feels at a loss** to reach you anymore, and is miserable over this.
- Your spouse feels that the "team" has been broken up and **is hurting** over this.
- Your spouse is **grieving the loss** of your parent to this disease, too.
- Your spouse is **as tired** as you are, especially if parenting and other responsibilities have been relegated to him.
- Your spouse **is only human**, and may selfishly (yet understandably) resent the intrusion of these problems in your lives.
- Your spouse **is still there**, which says a lot.

If you are thinking to yourself at this point, "Why should I think about **his** position when I'm the one with the problem?" then I strongly urge you to reconsider your point of view. Your problems are your spouse's and vice versa, and unless you have a commitment to working as a team you will continue to forge a stubborn, independent path that will likely destroy your partner's respect for you and your union. You have already veered off course and you must regain that cooperative spirit that you and your spouse need in order to be work together again and face this problem with clear heads, renewed energy and a sense of solidarity.

TAKE ACTION AND FEEL BETTER!

There are actions you can take to immediately release tension and restore harmonious feelings between you and your spouse.

- **Thank your partner** for the good things that he has provided during this time (a home for Grandpa, working hard to enable you to stay at home, doing carpool duty, meals, etc).
- **Let your spouse know** that while you will continue to honor your parent, you will give your marriage top priority in your life.
- **Tell your mate** you appreciate his input and want him involved in reviewing the best choices for a logical next step.
- **Inform your spouse** that the two of you will plan a getaway as soon as your parent is settled. Set a definitive date and keep it, even if it is simply for a night or two at a local hotel.
- **Let your spouse know** how much you value his support through this hard time.
- **Dream a little** and share your goals for the two of you, as well as your family. Include your parent when it is feasible.
- **Commit to** planned family and "date" nights. Mark them on the calendar with the letters "FUN" written in red ink.
- **Prioritize "time out"** intervals on a regular weekly basis – i.e., a solitary walk, breakfast in bed, or a shopping trip. Indulge yourself and you'll find yourself feeling more peaceful and easier to be around!

- **Re-establish traditions** with holiday get-togethers, family dinners, church-going, reading the paper at the table together, outings to sporting events. Schedule other commitments around these important rituals and stick with it.
- **Reward yourself** occasionally with a treat – a long, uninterrupted bath, a special dinner out, a massage or manicure, a drive along the shore or in the country, window-shopping, an evening with close friends, a matinee movie on a weekday.

Your spouse will see a balanced individual, who, while busy with life's cares, exhibits healthy boundaries, likes herself and is therefore better able to understand her own needs and those of her family. You will see a person who has discovered that admitting weakness is the first step towards gaining strength. And you'll both discover that it's much easier for two to circle a "bully" (problem) than it is for one to have to fight alone.

5

SIBLING RIVALRY

(What To Do When You Can't Agree)

L ET'S SAY THAT YOU know your parent is in trouble, a change is necessary, and everyone agrees, with the exception of one person – your sibling. Perhaps this sibling is the one who holds the purse strings or is "in charge" of your parent.

This chapter will explore how you can learn to handle this to your advantage.

Here's a sample of the types of concerns of family members:

"I agree something needs to be done, but my brother will flip out if we move mom. He can't believe what's happening. He's 3000 miles away and lives in a dream world. Mom always spoiled him."

"I don't get it – my sister's not stupid – in fact, she was picked to be mom's conservator because she's an attorney. But mom's falling apart and she won't do anything about it."

So what ***do*** you do if your sibling is unwilling to face facts? How do you enlist his cooperation without starting a fight? Do you just avoid the person entirely and hope he doesn't find out how you handle Mom's affairs? What power do you have if the other person has financial control or power of attorney designation? Can anything be done when the person is in charge but isn't exercising good judgment? What if your sibling is in denial that anything is wrong and wants you to mind your own business?

Yes, you can usually influence the course of care your parent receives even if your sibling has the authority but is doing nothing to ensure your parent is getting what she needs. You simply have to know how to do it.

It's discouraging when we feel we are shouldering a burden and yet feel powerless because of an uncooperative sibling. Before you lose your temper or create more animosity, try to realize that one of several things may be happening which may explain your sibling's avoidance of the dementia.

- **Your sibling is in denial** ("Maybe it will go away"). This emotional response is very common and is not a reflection of the person's intelligence or character.
- **Your sibling is afraid of the disease** ("Could it happen to me?"). In addition, your sibling may find the subject distasteful and/or the parent's weakness unsettling.
- **Your sibling is uneducated** about the severity of the disease and thinks it is part of the aging process. This response frequently accompanies denial.
- **Your sibling has distanced himself** enough to not be faced with the daily ravages of the disease and thus does not recognize the reality of the decline. Physical separation and infrequent visits have allowed the sibling to think the disease is under control.
- **Your sibling may hold unresolved anger** at past issues, such as resenting a parent's alcoholism, neglect,

or perceived favoritism of another child. This may have resulted in a need to "punish" the parent by now overlooking his needs.

- **Your sibling holds feelings of guilt** ("I should have paid more attention to her when she was well – I can't face her now") is a typical response. This belief fuels the person's insecurities about her ability or right to effect a change.
- **Concurrent personal problems** such as work pressures, illness, or marital difficulties provide a legitimate distraction (or excuse) for procrastination.
- **Burnout** from years of caring for parent can stall the problem-solving process.
- **Fear of change** ("What if I make the wrong decision?") can bring to a halt even the most simple of decisions in regards to helping an ailing parent.
- **Greed/Sense of entitlement** ("I deserve that house – if Mom sells it I'll get nothing") affects the direction of all care decisions. Adult children who value preservation of their inheritance over procuring quality care for their parents cannot be trusted to make good choices; the "bottom line" will rule in all deliberations.

In cases where families suspect or know of deliberate dishonesty or neglect on the part of an appointed conservator, it is necessary to take legal measures beginning with advice from a family law attorney to attempt to have a judge review the evidence and determine to revoke the appointment. However, when no criminal activity has occurred, most families do not need to resort to drastic measures. They simply need to be educated, purposeful and prepared to convincingly persuade the unwilling sibling to exercise sound judgment in helping move the parent from the present precarious arrangement to a better one. This chapter will outline suggestions on how to do this.

SUSPEND YOUR EMOTIONS

You've probably gathered by now that this book is not for the faint of heart. Over and over you will be required to put your own feelings aside and operate in a practical, calm manner. You will often need to suspend your emotions, kowtow, role-play, detach yourself, and utilize every diplomatic skill you can muster. I promise, though, that the self-control you will gain will make it all worth it. You will also be amazed at how much strength you have and how good it feels to be able to navigate these turbulent waters until you find a safe shore.

ATTITUDE ADJUSTMENT

The first thing you must do is to **develop an impartial attitude.** This is obviously not as easy as it sounds, but it is key to your success. No matter how annoying your sibling's actions are, you must view him with the calm detachment of an outsider. Pretend you are a paid consultant who has been retained to handle this matter.

These phrases are useful in helping alter your mindset. Steel yourself and repeat until memorized:

- **I will maintain a neutral attitude** towards my sibling.
- **I will behave in a professional manner** while dealing with this.
- **I will view this as a challenge** that I am capable of facing.
- **I will not allow my feelings to interfere** with my goal of a successful outcome.
- **I will suspend all judgment** and concentrate only on seeing this process through to a good end.
- **I will reach outside myself** to empathize with my sibling's position.
- **I can see this as my opportunity** to right some old wrongs with the power that I have.

- **This is my chance** to give to my family and learn some self-control.
- **I will be a better person** for it.
- **All that matters at this point** is that we get the help we need for our parent.

For some people this will require tremendous restraint in dealing with a relative, particularly if there has been a lifetime of tension in the relationship. Perhaps there has been favoritism shown towards a sibling, and that knowledge still hurts. You may be smarting because you should have been chosen to handle your parent's affairs, but were unfairly overlooked due to the sibling's positioning in family, gender, dominant personality, or financial power. Perhaps this sibling has made a mess of things, and as far as you are concerned, has a long history of screwing up, while you, the dutiful Cinderella, have always cleaned up after him.

GIVING LEADS TO RECEIVING

Comfort yourself by knowing that you may be completely correct in your assessment and justified in your feelings, but remind yourself that this point is really not of any consequence – and now that your parent is in the throes of the disease, you will likely never get the acknowledgment to which you feel entitled. However, you **will** receive great self-satisfaction by conducting yourself nobly and cleverly as you bring about positive change in your parent's care, and the greatest healing comes from sacrificial gestures. You may or may not be closer to your sibling down the line, but you will be surprised at how much self-respect you will gain. I know because I have witnessed this process time and again. Keep on!

BUILDING YOUR CASE

Now that you have some perspective on the need for detachment, it is time to begin building your case. Even if your sibling has no legal control over your parent, it is courteous and wise to involve him in the decisions involving care choices (unless the person is dangerous or unable/unwilling to be in contact). You may wonder why – if the person is marginally involved anyway, you should complicate things by bringing a sibling into the fold. Wouldn't it be easier to not have to weigh in that person's thoughts or wishes?

It is my opinion that unless your parent is in the end stages of the disease, you want as many advocates as possible in your corner, and most siblings usually reach a point of agreement despite rocky starts. Care for a parent who may have a significant number of years to live should ideally be a shared responsibility. If there is any possibility to forge a working relationship with family members, do it. Your parent needs back-up in the event that you are unable to intervene, and relatives are usually best suited to represent the person as they have an intimate understanding of the person. You deserve to have the comfort of knowing that another informed relative can step in and shoulder responsibility as needed.

If this is not possible, seek assistance from a trusted friend or other advocate. You will rest more easily if you know you have allies in your corner, and the burden will feel much lighter. You may in the course of time have a series of issues to face, and the more teamwork and cooperation you have, the better – especially if you have to deal with bureaucratic problems, personnel challenges, and other stressors.

GATHER YOUR FACTS

Since you are now prepared to handle the matter impartially, you must assemble your facts so they can be presented to your sibling. Get your notepad and start documenting **everything.** Gather evidence that shows that your parent is in need of more help. You can:

- **Drop in unannounced** at various times of day and night. Stagger your visits and record the times. Write down your findings, for example: "Food with mold, Dad unshaven, bathtub bone dry, house filthy, clothing worn backwards, fearful of intruders, stove burner left on, parent uncharacteristically angry – screamed at cat."
- **Record all dates and times**. Be specific. Don't write impressions – just note the facts. Get corroboration, feedback and quotes from neighbors, social workers, delivery or mail carriers. Poll friends of your parents.
- **Accompany** parent for check-up or arrange for public health nurse to stop by. Set up meal delivery with Meals on Wheels or similar service. You will receive additional support for your case when your parent receives an assessment by a nurse or social worker. Ask your parent's doctor for a written statement outlining recommendations. (He won't release confidential medical information but will usually consent to accommodate your request with a note highlighting potential risks that his patient is currently facing).
- **Contact** your local ombudsman for a meeting. These are volunteer advocates who can help you in evaluating your parent. They can also recommend programs in your area. Document your appointment.
- **Assemble** literature from the Alzheimer's Association, adult day programs, and care facilities.
- **Call or visit** the Area Office on Aging. Stock up on brochures.
- **Set up tours** of local facilities and programs. Visit a geriatric psychiatry program at participating hospitals.
- **Contact** Adult Protective Services (if the domestic situation is life-threatening to your parent). An investigation and home visit will be conducted and a report filed. Request a copy for your family conference.

When a parent is a danger to himself or others you must notify your sibling and inform him of this possibility. Even if you have predicted this crisis, act as though this is a sudden surprise. There is no point in angrily rebuking your sibling for being asleep at the wheel. You'll get nowhere and will only put the person on the defensive. Use an assumptive tone and convey the attitude that you're sure your sibling is unaware of how bad the situation is. Behave as though shocked, but in control. Otherwise, your sibling may react as though you are blaming him for the crisis and inferring that this happened under his nose. If this happens, he will resist your help and possibly stall or subvert the process. Come alongside your sibling and put your plan in action.

BRING IN REINFORCEMENTS

As the book of Proverbs puts it, "Without the counsel of others, people will fall, but there is wisdom in the multitude of counselors." Prudent people realize the value of seeking objective input to aid in clear-headed decision-making. Now is the time to get your backup team ready! Align yourself with relatives, physician, pastor or rabbi, good family friends, social workers, and anyone else who can support you in your quest to overcome the roadblock you are facing. Explain that you will need to convince your sibling of the severity of the problem and will require these peoples' assistance. Do **not** position yourself as an adversary to your sibling, as people may feel reluctant to be drawn into what could be viewed as a family feud. Quietly discuss with your support base your deep concerns for your parent's health and your belief that the matter seems to be too overwhelming for your sibling, who may not have all the facts. Tell them you would like to arrange a family conference and the presence of impartial outsiders would help greatly to keep the meeting objective and focused on developing an action plan. Share any updates on your parent's condition to bolster your case.

Once you have enlisted the support of others, contact your sibling and respectfully share that recent critical developments have necessitated a family council, either by conference call (if distances are an issue) or in a meeting at your home. Keep it on your own turf if at all possible, as you will feel more secure psychologically. Be calm and assumptive, with an attitude of concern and inclusiveness.

Some siblings may balk, which is why you want to have your evidence compiled and at hand. Once you've corroborated your suspicions with medical reports, testimony from neighbors, friends and others, share with your sibling a bit of it. For example: "Pat, I was just notified by mom's neighbor that she was ringing doorbells last night up and down the block. The police were called and a social worker will follow up in a few days. I'd like us to brainstorm before then so we can be ready, and also protect mom from doing this again. Dr. Barnes has some recommendations he faxed to me and Nancy and Jim can be at the house by 7:00. We'll certainly wait until you can get here, because we need your thoughts and ideas, too."

Share with your relative that your observations about your parent have been backed up by concerned friends and professionals, (in case your sibling protests that the current problem is an isolated incident). Explain that the current situation is no longer working and if more convincing is needed, cite concrete examples that you have already documented. Be specific and don't dramatize.

If your sibling still refuses to meet, inform him that any further delays could prove harmful to your parent and that the next step means the involvement of Adult Protective Services. Tell him that in good conscience you cannot remain inactive knowing that your parent is at risk for accident, injury or distress. Speak calmly and keep it impersonal, even if you are infuriated. You have presented your case well and have demonstrated that you have a network of supporters who are aware of the situation. In a nice way, you are reminding your sibling that you have evidence and people to back you. Usually at this point even the most stubborn family members will realize that you are not to be dissuaded, and will consent to meet. Because they have been avoiding the problem, they often have no contingency plan of their own, and will usually be open to your suggestions. Remember, their resistance usually reflects emotional unwillingness, not differences of philosophy.

Be sensitive and ask if it would be preferable for you to make all care arrangements on his behalf. Let him know that you are willing to do all the legwork in visiting facilities, interviewing caregivers, or meeting with doctors, but that you will always keep him abreast of significant changes, health updates, and other pertinent information. You'll also ensure that he receives any documentation requiring his attention or signature. He'll get the picture.

Only in the most extreme cases do family members need to threaten to have the POA (power of attorney) designation revoked. This is a last resort that must be implemented if the sibling fails to agree with or offer a viable plan of care to protect the senior. This scenario will likely not occur, as most siblings usually behave reasonably once they accept the fact that the problem is not going away and that you are clear in your commitment to resolve the matter.

HOST A FAMILY COUNCIL

Now you have your data on paper, your support team in your home, and your sibling arrives. Console yourself that you are in good company and try to empathize with your sibling, who may be feeling a bit railroaded. As you begin the meeting, determine to show grace, even if you still feel that your sibling is being un-realistic or childish.

SHOULD IT GET PERSONAL?

Some professionals counsel families not to use a family council to delve into personal issues, but I have found that this is often necessary in order to move past stubborn resistance and reach the goal of re-establishing relationships and fostering cooperation. It is correct, though, not to allow much time to be spent airing old issues, as things can digress and get out of hand if not properly mediated. Deep-rooted thought patterns won't be changed overnight, and the sibling can certainly seek out more in-depth counseling at a later date to analyze his issues comprehensively. The objective here is to remove the barrier of unwillingness and reach a mutual understanding that the family must be in one accord in tackling the parent's dementia. This can often be achieved if you allow a resentful sibling an opportunity to share, and if you acknowledge the hurt. I have seen this act of sensitivity work wonders in helping the person feel less adversarial and thus be able to drop the defenses. This enables everyone to re-focus on the challenge at hand.

Your sibling may need to blow off steam. If you sense this, prepare to let him do that. Sometimes the person has years of pent-up jealousy, anger, and other complex emotions that are now compounded by the unhappiness of dealing with this additional burden. Don't let things become maudlin, but do allow the person a chance to share his feelings. If you do this, you will have gone a long way towards clearing the air and winning the respect of your relative. Keep it brief, but encourage the sibling to talk. Apologize if you need to. Offer to give whatever support you can from here on. You will be amazed to witness how far a little humility goes in restoring relationships. You might also find empathy that you did not feel before, and even some fresh insight into your sibling's position that was not there before.

WATCH YOUR LANGUAGE

I have sat through many family councils, and while the members may be sophisticated, bright, good people, the emotional tension can run high. This can be avoided by use of inclusive language spoken sensitively.

Bridges are not only made of wood or steel, but of words, as well. Some people are naturally gifted in diplomacy, while the rest of us have to work on honing this skill. Start by thinking about the impact of your words and stretch yourself by carefully controlling your speech that will draw in your sibling.

*What **Not** To Say:*

"We have to handle Mother whether you like it or not!"
-or-
*"Why do **I** always have to bring these things up?"*

Try Instead:

"I know you love Mom a lot, and I'm sure you and Sue are as worried as we are"
-or-
"I'm sure you've noticed the decline – I'm so glad we can figure this out together."

TIPS TO REMEMBER

Your "word bridges" will signal to your sibling that you are an ally.

Think of how you can use language to bond instead of divide. Not only will this kind gesture help you ace this meeting, it will serve you well in all of your interpersonal relations. I have seen screaming matches between adversarial siblings begin *or* end based on the words chosen and spoken. Stay in control.

Keep in mind these helpful hints:

- **Resolve** not to raise your voice under any circumstances.
- **Validate** the contribution (even if all he's done is come to the council) that the person has made.
- **Demonstrate** a desire to work things out by offering to handle the most difficult tasks needed in the transitional period of preparing a care plan.
- **Catch loaded phrases** and avoid saying words like "always" and "never."
- **Sincerely compliment** the person's efforts – "I know you've held this together a long time. Thank you."
- **Affirm** what the person says, with statements like "I know" and "I think I understand."
- **Focus** on parent and his needs. Do not allow yourself to stray from this, except to briefly acknowledge emotion.

INCLUSIVE PHRASES

- "**I know** you've shouldered this for a long time. I'm glad I can offer you more help."
- "**I'm sorry** I was so wrapped up in my own life. I didn't understand."
- "**You're right** – she doesn't deserve our help, but I like to think we're not like her."
- "**It must have been tough** being head of the family when you were just a teenager."
- "**I don't blame you** for not wanting to help Dad. I'd feel the same way if I went through what you did."
- "**I know** how close you've always been to them, and how hard this must be."
- "**Thank you** for everything you've done."
- "Her alcoholism **was the worst** thing in my life, too."
- "**I need** your help."
- "**Thanks for being willing** to hear me out. I appreciate it more than you know."

- "**I choose** to see her as pathetic. It helps me to think that way and let the past go."

Language like this and attentive listening goes a long way towards easing tensions between siblings. Once you have constructed your bridge, you may cross it together.

CROSSING TO THE OTHER SIDE

By establishing a link with your sibling, you can expect to see the resistance lessen and a growing ability to dialogue about your parent. At this point introduce your findings and set a plan in place. Explain that circumstances dictate an immediate plan of action and present your information on available resources. Give everyone in attendance an opportunity to speak and consider each person's input. You'll be pleased to find a spirit of cooperation and hear some good ideas, too, as you review the available options and vote on a plan of care.

6

CONVINCING THE CAREGIVING SPOUSE

ONE OF MY CLIENTS, Susan S., shared with me her thoughts:

"I can't believe my dad. Here he is, 85 years old, with a heart problem, and he won't ask for help with mom. He almost fell with her on top of him when he tried to get her in the car yesterday! I don't even know how he's able to bathe her, in fact, it's happening less frequently because I've noticed her hair isn't always clean like it used to be."

When asked if she had expressed her concerns to her father, Susan replied, "Well, I've tried, but Dad just gets annoyed and says he's fine. I know he's not, but he won't admit it."

A JOB WITH NO BREAKS

Caring for a spouse afflicted with dementia is an exhausting, ever-changing task. Each new day brings different challenges. In addition to dealing with the physical and emotional needs of the patient, the spouse through it all must come to grips with the changing nature of the relationship and face the fact that the partnership the couple once had is forever altered.

Many caregivers have wearily likened the experience to having a newborn infant in the house again, albeit without a supportive partner and considerably diminished energy. Caregiving spouses face a lonely, 24-hour job that offers no perks or even the consolation of solace and companionship from co-workers. In fact, there are no break periods – just snatched moments in which to run to the bathroom or grab a sandwich when their charge is distracted or sleeping.

So with home care, adult day programs, specialized facilities and support services a-plenty, why is it so difficult to convince an overburdened caregiver that it is time to seek out help? Why do logical, intelligent people position themselves so precariously? Why do they take risks that they would discourage others from acting on? Why do they wait so long to admit they can't operate under this burden? And why are they so embarrassed to concede that they desperately need help?

Of course, there may be other reasons that a caregiver chooses to procrastinate, or perhaps you may be frustrated that the person claims to not know why he chooses to dither. It is usually easy to figure out why the person is stuck if you can determine what his biggest fear is. Compliment him or her on their devotion to their spouse and be genuine in inquiring of them what their utmost concerns are. Choose a moment when the person is not overwrought and defensive, and you'll get your answer.

RED FLAGS SIGNAL BURNOUT

If a caregiver can honestly answer three or more of the following questions with a "yes," he/she is in danger of burnout and the problems associated with it. Familiarize yourself with the questions so that you can discuss them sensitively with the caregiver at the proper time.

- Am I finding myself more and more fearful of an accident occurring in the home?
- Am I letting family/friends see a rosier picture of the senior than really is the case?
- Am I growing to resent my spouse's demands? Do I feel like lashing out at him occasionally or frequently?
- Am I too embarrassed to take him out in public (church, restaurant) for fear of his unpredictability? Am I resentful of what we're missing?
- Have I neglected my own health (no time or energy for exercise or breaks)?
- Have I stopped taking much-needed respite (a night or weekend away while spouse stays with trusted caregivers or family)? Do I trust that anyone else can do the job?
- Have I risked injury doing lifting, bathing, transferring to a wheelchair, and other arduous tasks? Am I too proud to admit that I do not have the strength to safely perform these tasks?
- Have I felt like coping with the aid of alcohol or tranquilizers? Does anybody suspect?
- Do I wish my spouse sometimes were dead and then feel evil for thinking such a thing?
- Do I feel that this is just my "lot in life" and should not make a big deal of it?
- Am I losing precious sleep coping with night wandering or other erratic behavior?
- Have I had to fend off a physical attack from my spouse?
- Have I had to fight with my spouse regularly to get him to eat, bathe or do other necessary things? Do I keep my cool or am I as upset as he at the end of the argument?
- Do I lie awake wondering what will happen if I die first?
- Am I increasingly tense compared to how I used to be?

- Do I consider my personality increasingly robotic and dull? Have I begun to feel that I am merely existing and not living?

If the caregiver answers three or more questions in the affirmative, it should serve as an alarm to all involved that the person is overwhelmed and at risk for physical or emotional breakdown. Family members reading this will generally have an accurate assessment of whether or not the caregiver is coping well and is overextended, and it is imperative that these warning signs are not dismissed.

Let's take a look at the reasons caregivers most often cite for delaying in getting the help they need before we examine how to begin laying a foundation for obtaining aid.

Some fears listed are legitimate, while some are a result of misconceptions, conditioning, or ignorance. At any rate, you will need to identify which issues are holding up your family member in order to prepare a useful response.

Of course, there may be other reasons that a caregiver chooses to procrastinate, or perhaps you may be frustrated that the person claims to not know why he won't seek help. It is usually easy to figure out why the person is stuck if you can determine what his biggest fear is. Compliment her on her devotion to her spouse and be genuine in inquiring of her about her utmost concerns. Choose a moment when the person is not overwrought and defensive, and you'll get your answer.

TOP TWELVE REASONS CAREGIVERS PROCRASTINATE:

Fear of losing identity. "I've always cared for your father's needs." Men and women who have devoted their entire married life to caring for the needs of their family (particularly those who eschewed careers or outside interests) may face tremendous apprehension that a new caretaker will usurp their role. These spouses need to learn the perspective that their role is not being *removed*, but merely altered. A good way to do this is to have a family conference actively involving the spouse by discussing his strengths ("You keep the most meticulous records," "No one can get Mom to laugh the way you can") and delegating specific duties that will help reinforce the spouse's sense of contribution while outside aid is being enlisted.

Fear of being misunderstood. "People will think I'm dumping him." Spouses who place great stock in the opinions of others need to be reminded that true friends do not second-guess serious decisions such as placement of a parent, but care about the welfare of the entire family.

Fear of manipulation. "If I get help, he'll yell, cry, and be such a pill – it's just easier to do it myself." Spouses who operate under this misconception are usually surprised to find out that well-trained professional caregivers often draw out the individual in a variety of positive ways. The senior often interprets the interaction as "having company" and will behave passively and politely under the proper direction.

Fear that resources will be exhausted. "We'll be wiped out if I get help." In this case, it is important to seek the counsel of specialists such as elder law and tax attorneys, financial planners, geriatric care managers, and other professionals who can educate families in obtaining financial assistance and utilizing existing resources. (See Chapter 8)

Deep-rooted belief that responsibility is solely the spouse's. "In sickness and in health." Some spouses feel they are disloyal and failing their partner if they admit that they cannot handle the demands of caring for them. They often react defensively to the well-meaning protests of others, justifying themselves by insisting that "no one understands" their traditional values. Best response – "You're right, Mom. I really admire how seriously you take your vows to Dad. People have gotten away from that type of commitment. In Grandma's day, you could count on a lot of community support rallying around someone who was ill. We kids want to do our share."

Cultural expectations. "It's expected in our family/culture to take in our grandparents." People who come from extended family structures (multiple generations living in one household) often face great pressure to continue this tradition, despite the fact that the needs of the aging parent are often far more serious than those their forebears likely encountered. An excellent option for these families is to seek out experienced home health aides who are from the same culture and could assimilate into the family structure with ease.

Stoicism. "I don't know why everyone is worried about it – I can handle it." This is a trait that is particularly common with retired males, who often reluctantly grapple with the physical limitations that aging brings. Families need to be sensitive to this and work with the caregiving parent by highlighting his strengths and formulating a plan of action that uses those assets while augmenting them with support services.

'Martyr' complex "This is my lot in life." The spouses I worked with who sported this philosophy were often the angriest people I ever counseled, despite their "poor little me" persona that they tried to project. These are individuals who often wield their power as victims, and have a lifelong pattern of doing this. Their family members see right through this and it is a source of tremendous tension usually. It is a very manipulative position to take, despite protestations by the person that he has no control over the situation. The person may deliberately refuse help as a form of punishment towards his ill spouse (although he would furiously deny this). I have often urged families who face this sort of resistance to seek medical assistance for the person by a competent physician skilled in handling depression. Start by encouraging the person to get a complete physical. Alert the family doctor with your concern and ask if he or she can discuss utilizing appropriate medications and therapy that can help.

Deep distrust of psychiatry/institutions/therapy. "No headshrinkers or nuthouses for our family!" This may occur in families with limited education or exposure to specialized forms of care and intervention. Some may be frightened at the possibility that they would be indirectly responsible for inflicting trauma on their loved one, while some people confuse dementia with mental illness (such as schizophrenia). Because they have little understanding of modern treatment programs, they do not realize how many options are available to them and how they can make informed decisions. Families can best help by de-stigmatizing dementia and educating the spouse about this medical condition, sharing literature and having the family physician discuss a course of action.

Denial in the permanency of the disease. "He always perks up in the morning." While it is true that dementia victims do have "clearer" days, the decline in most cases is imminent and there is no cure or return to normalcy. The sooner the spouse comes to understand this the sooner she can begin to prepare herself for the changes that accompany each stage of the disease. Support groups (see Chapter 7) are wonderful aids in helping the individual come to grips with this.

Fear of hastening the inevitable. "If I move him, he will die." Caregivers should be aware of the statistics that reveal a high number of mates actually predecease their ill spouse (the inference is that they have neglected their own health). Spouses also need to know that unless the person is moved unnecessarily (in the midst of serious illness, into a facility that gives poor care, etc.) he will likely begin to show some degree of stability and often *improvement* as a result of three square meals, stimulation and good care. The physician can help by arranging to monitor the progress of the patient, thus allaying the spouse's fears.

Resentment/insecurity at new role. "Dad always planned everything." The spouse who has been thrust into a new role as sole decision-maker may feel woefully inadequate, particularly if the partner was the driving force throughout the course of the relationship. Families can aid the person by discussing this ("I know Dad's dementia was the last thing you could have expected for your retirement years") and reassuring the spouse that she is not alone with this challenge.

LAYING A FOUNDATION

Once you have a clear idea of *why* the caregiver may be procrastinating in getting help, you will know which hurdle must be overcome and begin to put together a plan of action. It is important not to gloss over the cause of the well spouse's indecision, because until you can acknowledge and understand it you will not be able to lovingly and creatively take the person by the arm and direct him down a path that will yield better results.

Position yourself carefully. Start by simply demonstrating your willingness to take on as many tasks as you are able. Resist the urge to criticize when you see questionable moves and respond tactfully rather than forcefully ("I haven't gotten any exercise all week, so why don't I help Dad into the shower so you can have a snack?") Cheerfully establish yourself as an ally and you'll soon win that person's confidences. At that point, you may safely introduce the subject of support services, beginning with the family physician (discussed in detail in Chapter 19).

TRANSITION AND THE CAREGIVER

In my meetings with families I would often mention to them that transitional periods following a move or significant change to their loved one's lifestyle would be harder, generally, on the caregiver than the senior – particularly as the disease became more advanced. As the dementia progresses, the person's sense of time becomes blurred and details that once would have been a source of concern cease to be a consideration. Many residents that I admitted to our facilities (provided that they passed the pre-qualification standard) adapted to their environment on average within the first month or so. The transition was fairly rapid simply because the residents' most basic needs were being met and the clients felt cared for.

Caregivers are usually fairly surprised to learn this, but relief accompanies this revelation, as most people are convinced that change is most traumatic for the ill person. A burden is lifted when the caregiver can redefine her role as **life partner**, not lifeline.

SHIFTING VALUES AND STANDARDS

It is important for caregivers, relatives and friends to remember that **their values significantly differ from those of the individual with dementia**. The person's most pressing needs (food, warmth, shelter, attention) replace the desire for material items, meaningful relationships, shared interests and other intangible values once held.

Families seeking to move a parent into a facility need not worry too much about "roommate matching" as one would in an independent apartment or retirement community. Providing that the roommate is not a behavioral challenge, most pairings are relatively peaceful and the cohabitation uneventful, as the senior is long past the point of being able to consider philosophical differences.

This shift offers relief to families, who begin to realize that their loved one is becoming more egocentric and childlike in his demands, only caring about **what** he needs and **when** it is needed. "Home" simply becomes wherever he is at the moment. *People with dementia live in the here and now.*

Once family members comprehend this, they are usually able to gain the perspective needed to realize that the dementia is multi-faceted and requires more resources than one person can offer.

A WORD OF CAUTION

Caregiving spouses *do* need to keep in mind that because their mates live largely in the moment and are now in the care of others it is possible for "romantic" attachments to form with fellow residents or other care providers. Most spouses understand that reasons for this can vary, sometimes simply because the object of affection is kindly or reminds the senior of the spouse or a former sweetheart. One lady I worked with was horrified to see her husband walking hand-in-hand with a woman in the community. Moreover, she was amazed at her husband's amicable manner, as she confided that her spouse had always been aloof and physically undemonstrative. She soon came to understand that the disease affected her husband's judgment and that his behavior was a result of this. However, staff should be sensitive to these issues in the event that spouses are troubled by special "friendships" and monitor them accordingly. Our management team learned that this was a topic that needed to be broached with families in advance, to spare the well spouse any unnecessary upset or surprises at visiting time.

Caregivers need to feel reinforced and supported by those around them. Family and friends should be encouraged to know that "stubborn" spouses are not as resolute as they appear; they simply have painted themselves into a corner and need a face-saving way to emerge. Your understanding will make all the difference to a tired caregiver.

At this point, you may wish to further assist the caregiver by accompanying her to a support group meeting in your area. The following chapter will outline this valuable service.

7

SUPPORT GROUPS

"I am here tonight because my husband will leave me if I don't find a place for Dad NOW. He's been living at my house this year and it's driving us crazy."

"I wish I were as wonderful as the rest of you (here in the support group). Truth be told, I can't stand being around my mother – and she's not a tyrant – in fact, she's very sweet. She just hovers around me! Frankly, I came here tonight just mainly to get away from her."

"I have so much guilt about moving my parents to a dementia facility. They were always so good to me. I feel like I'm dumping them. I'm so tired of this."

"My husband refuses to help. He resents that mom and dad frittered away their money and made no plans for the future."

Men and women attending support group meetings are able to vent their feelings in a safe, non-judgmental environment. Comments such as the above stated ones are a common sampling of the types of concerns that attendees face and discuss.

Volunteer, trained facilitators sponsored by the Alzheimer's Association and other organizations preside over group meetings. Most sessions convene monthly or bi-monthly. The objective is to provide families a safe forum in which to freely share thoughts, feelings, and even fears. Support and information are readily available, and attendees are encouraged to bring the senior if the person is fairly functional (early stages) and would not disrupt the group or walk away. However, since the purpose of the meeting is to help the individual sort his thoughts, it would be counterproductive to bring a severely confused family member.

WHO SHOULD ATTEND A SUPPORT GROUP?

Anyone who is facing the challenges of caring for a person with dementia, or is acquainted with a family struggling with the disease would benefit from the knowledge gained at a support group meeting. I have attended support group meetings and have been gratified to see a variety of individuals from different walks of life gathered together sharing, listening, and sometimes crying. I've interacted with ex-wives, friends, spouses, relatives, service providers, and even young children who have come together in an atmosphere of support and acceptance to learn how to better cope with this malady.

One woman brought along her nine-year old daughter to a meeting. After the adults in the circle commiserated, the facilitator gently asked the girl if she was interested in talking about how she felt about her grandmother (who had dementia). With some quiet encouragement from her mother, the child admitted that her feelings were hurt "when Grandma yells at me."

At this point, the ice was broken and the girl continued to explain her bewilderment about grandmother's unpredictable behavior and frequent outbursts. The facilitator adeptly helped the child understand that the *disease* was the culprit – that it was the dementia snapping (not grandmother). The girl seemed to be able to grasp this truth, and became calmer as she digested this information and listened to others' stories.

WHERE DO SUPPORT GROUPS MEET?

Support group meetings are usually held once a month and are sponsored by various churches, assisted living facilities, senior centers, hospitals and the like. The Alzheimer's Association provides training and materials free of charge to the public. You may contact the Alzheimer's Association or go online to find out meeting dates, times and locations. Your local newspaper will also likely list this information in its community events' section. Don't forget to consult your senior resource guide, your area Office on Aging and local above-mentioned institutions for meeting details. With the exception of those who live in remote rural areas, most people can easily access regular meetings.

BENEFITS OF SUPPORT GROUPS

Some of the many benefits support groups offer include:

- Trained, professional coordinators who monitor protocol and direction of meeting in order to keep session moving in a productive and orderly fashion.
- Up-to-date resources, literature, and practical tips are disbursed with advice ranging from caregiving hints to handling difficult behaviors, communication guidelines, medical and legislative updates, and other useful information. Members often recommend books and other professional tools that have proven helpful, particularly for newcomers who need to learn as much as they can about the disease.

- Impartial, non-judgmental facilitation and acceptance.
- A sense of empathy from others facing similar challenges.
- A safe forum to express anger, confide frustration and needs.
- An opportunity to give or receive valuable input.
- Discreet formats (similar to "anonymous" groups like AA). Confidentiality is respected.
- A structured setting with observed protocol, which allows even flow of information and prevents one person from dominating conversation.
- Time set aside for specific problem solving of current dilemmas.
- A needed "break" for caregivers.

Support groups can't make problems vanish, but they will help a person feel less isolated during this trying time. I especially recommend these meetings to be suggested to family members struggling with denial or confused about the changes they are encountering. Most people are less resistant to receiving advice from a source outside of the family. An informed, impartial facilitator is usually more credible to an upset family member than even the most knowledgeable sibling. This may seem unfair, but a discerning individual will realize that the main objective is to get the help needed – **now**.

Support group meetings have often been catalysts for helping reluctant family members face facts and begin to consider enlisting the aid of physicians, service professionals and others who can help bring about relief and change to a desperate situation.

8

COMMUNITY RESOURCES

S O HOW DOES ONE find out sources of help in the community? The good news is that there is an abundance of information readily available! There are various avenues a person can access to gather information, including:

THE INTERNET – There are websites for facilities, support groups, service organizations, research data, and up-to-date information on dementia/Alzheimer's disease, and related topics.

PRINT MEDIA – Books, resource guides and magazines are plentiful. There are free periodicals offering financial and legal advice, and referral guides (small magazines distributed through doctor's offices, senior centers and other services providers). These mini-directories offer a comprehensive listing of facilities, agencies, adult day programs, and service providers.

GOVERNMENT AGENCIES – Veteran's Affairs, Area Agency on Aging and the Department of Social Services have local listings and offices, as well as representatives who will help you with your inquiry. You can call information for toll-free or local branch office numbers, or set an appointment to meet with a counselor. For emergency information, call Adult Protective Services or dial 911.

Most cities have an entire community service department that offers programs for all citizens. Ask to speak to the director of senior services or a representative who serves as a liaison for that population. This person often serves as the manager of the local senior center.

Many cities today host a monthly senior "roundtable" meeting at the senior center. Area professionals gather to discuss pertinent legislation and senior topics and to network with one another. If you attend these open meetings you will be able to meet and share with an array of service providers. Call to find out when and where these sessions are held.

MEDICAL PROFESSIONALS – Check your local newspaper to learn about lectures featuring geriatric specialists sponsored by hospitals and senior facilities. These events are usually free to the public and very informative.

- *Parish nurses* render a relatively new service sponsored by many churches. These programs are staffed by volunteers or paid professionals using their nursing skills to serve the community. Arrange to speak with the director of the program.
- *Visiting nurses* are contracted when you call your local Visiting Nurse Association and arrange for an evaluation and home visit.
- *Geriatric psychiatrists and inpatient programs* are available in most states (see Chapter 9). Check your telephone listings or contact your HMO or health care provider for names of physicians and psychologists trained

in senior mental health. If your medical program requires you to obtain a referral first, be politely persistent and do what it takes to accomplish this.

- **Social workers** are another source of valuable information. If you belong to a certain medical plan, check your directory for a listing of social workers and case managers, or try a local nursing home. Conscientious social workers take a sincere interest in the welfare of their patients and are familiar with local facilities and the quality of care provided. They are also usually well-acquainted with hospice, home health, and other services, as well as Medicare and aid programs.

LEGAL RESOURCES – Your phone book has listings of attorneys who specialize in elder laws, wills, trusts and related matters. You may also contact your local American Bar Association chapter for additional referrals. Because "elder law" is a rather broad term, it is important to find an attorney who has experience with the specific area you need help in – i.e., Medicare claims and appeals, disability planning, durable power of attorney, elder abuse and fraud recovery, estate planning, health law, long-term care placements, etc.

CLERGY – Many religious organizations offer ministries to senior citizens. See if your place of worship offers this service and talk to the senior liaison. Try your local hospital chaplain, as well. Such ministers are usually happy to share about local resources and may offer counsel as needed.

SENIOR ADVOCATES & SERVICE ORGANIZATIONS – You may arrange to receive newsletters and other pertinent information by contacting the Alzheimer's Association in your area. This organization has offices nationwide and is an outstanding source of articles and information on facilities, support groups and resources.

- The **American Association of Retired Persons (AARP)** has a nationwide network offering information on everything from identity theft, safe driving and consumer tips for seniors, in addition to valuable updates on legislation and initiatives that may impact the disabled elderly. Stay informed.
- **Meals On Wheels** – There are chapters in most cities of this low-cost meal program for homebound seniors. Senior centers contract with these and other agencies that offer these services. Check your telephone directory for a listing, or call your nearest senior center.
- **Geriatric care managers** work for private agencies and will assess your family member's needs and recommend a course of action for home care. These professionals are usually trained in gerontology, social work, or nursing and are a good source of assistance especially for families who live out of the area.
- **Referral agencies** are organizations that offer to help you find placement or assistance for your loved one. The service is free, based upon information that you provide on the resident's need, budget and locale. They will forward your request to facilities that seem to be good candidates for consideration. The facility will in turn contact you.

The referral agency has a contractual arrangement with nursing homes, assisted living and board and care facilities, and receives a finder's fee from the facility should placement occur. Larger referral facilities maintain a listing of thousands of facilities and agencies statewide. These agencies can also help place clients who desire a facility that caters to a particular ethnic/religious persuasion, or have other special needs.

Look online or in your phone book for a listing of referral agencies in your state or region. You will want to choose an agency that routinely (at least, annually) visits and evaluates facilities.

Legitimate agencies will take an active interest in referring to reputable businesses only.

Of course, you will still need to thoroughly investigate all leads. Facilities and care management can be adversely affected by changes in management. You may receive a glowing recommendation about a facility or service provider that is now declining due to new management.

Before determining a course of care, you may wish to investigate a reputable senior mental health program in your area, particularly if the senior is demonstrating increasingly alarming/ uncharacteristic behavior. It is important for this problem to be addressed and proper treatment sought prior to effecting a significant lifestyle change. The following chapter will explore geriatric psychiatry and outline the services offered.

9

SENIOR MENTAL HEALTH ("GERO-PSYCH") PROGRAMS

MANY HOSPITALS TODAY OFFER programs for seniors who can be admitted for psychiatric observation and support. These programs are commonly nicknamed "Gero (Geriatric) Psych" and refer to the treatment of mature adults who exhibit one or more of the following symptoms:

- Withdrawn behavior
- Confusion/Disorientation
- Sleep disorders
- Agitation
- Depression
- Paranoia
- Erratic patterns
- Depleted energy/lethargy
- Persistent anger/sadness
- Inability to function in activities of daily living

BENEFITS OF A GERO-PSYCH PROGRAM

Many families and caregivers of seniors admitted to gero-psych programs support these services as they have seen distressing behaviors curbed thanks to medical intervention, family counseling, and individual and group therapy. These programs benefit qualified patients because they offer daily monitoring by geriatric psychiatrists who work closely with the patient and medical team to help develop coping skills and address psychiatric symptoms (which positively affects physical status as well).

The goal of this program, in a nutshell, is to help stabilize behavior so that the senior can resume functioning with the social and life skills necessary at home or in a community setting. Some residents have utilized the program's services more than once over the course of several years, as needed.

Some families measure success of the program in different ways – primarily in terms of behavioral changes, most notably as they witness the senior gaining more emotional calm and equilibrium. Some families are grateful to the program for helping the patient feel an added sense of security from a perceived sense of "importance" (particularly if the person had lived a very lonely, isolated life prior to admission). "I think Mom liked all the attention she got from the nurses," was a comment I heard on more than one occasion. "She ate every meal and even put on weight!" was another observation.

For family members who may be in denial about the seriousness of the dementia, the interaction with the psych team will help convince the person of the reality of the disease. An inpatient stay in such a program can help family members align with the medical staff to help present to the reluctant caregiver a positive plan of action post-discharge.

WHO QUALIFIES FOR THE PROGRAM?

According to Mina Spadaro, clinical director of West Anaheim Medical Center's Renewal Behavioral Health program, admission to these programs is dependent upon several variables. Essentially, to enter an inpatient program, a patient must be an adult over the age of 40 who has exhibited self-destructive behaviors towards himself or others. Patients enter the program of their own volition or with the consent of a conservator or power of attorney who has specific designation to make mental health decisions. "While we do admit those who suffer acute agitation that may be a threat to themselves or others, we do not accept 5150* designees," Ms. Spadaro explained.

Admission Criteria (2006) for the program outlines who can be admitted into the program with three categories – **threat to self** (whether overt, as in suicidal behavior, or *"chronic and continuing self-destructive behavior that poses a significant and/ or immediate threat to life, limb or bodily function*; **threat to others,** defined in part as *"assaultive behavior, major disability in social, interpersonal, occupational and or educational functioning that is leading to dangerous or life-threatening function,* **or** *"mental disorder causing an inability to maintain adequate nutrition or self-care."* Many patients that fall into the latter category are admitted into the program.

The third criterion for admission is **failure of outpatient psychiatric treatment**, which may occur due to "increasing severity of psychiatric symptoms and inadequate clinical response to psychotropic medications." Sometimes an extended, inpatient program where patients can experience close monitoring can make all the difference in the treatment of maladaptive behaviors.

---

* In the state of California, a legal hold that is imposed on a person believed to be in need of psychiatric treatment.

WHO WOULD NOT QUALIFY?

Because the program is designed to help stabilize behaviors through medication monitoring and therapy, it would not be appropriate to admit patients who have a dementia diagnosis absent of acute behavioral change or with no expectation of a positive response to treatment. In other words, mild confusion or early stage dementia **without** accompanying behavioral disorders does not qualify a patient for admittance.

It is also necessary that the patient consent to participate in the program and has a primary psychiatric diagnosis. In other words, the program will not admit someone who "needs a home" due to an unrelated disorder, as a substitute for incarceration, or because they are being treated for medical problems but are "difficult" patients.

Patients with terminal or life-threatening diseases or in need of complex medical or surgical procedures do not qualify, but the program can help those who do have medical conditions that include the need for oxygen, IV's, dialysis, or walking devices and wheelchairs.

WHO PAYS FOR IT?

In most cases, Medicare will cover the costs of an inpatient stay, usually for up to a period of fourteen days, "although in our Renewal program we have kept patients over for several additional days if need be," asserted Ms. Spadaro. Some families opt to pay cash at a daily rate for treatment. Date of discharge is determined based up how well the patient has responded to medications and therapy.

STAFFING

The first point of contact at time of admission is usually the social worker, head nurse or director of the program. Families need to provide a list of current medications, insurance information, and other pertinent data. A care plan is individualized to each patient; it will include the assignment of a team including care/coordinators, recreation therapists, psychiatric nurses, psychiatrists and other physicians to the case. Most patients occupy shared living quarters within a secured area of the hospital.

ROUTINE

A typical day begins with breakfast between 7:00 and 8:00, group therapy and sporadic rest and activity times, punctuated by physician visits and meetings. Medications are adjusted and monitored and family visits are permitted according to hospital guidelines. Caregivers are free to contact the director for regular updates on the patient's condition, and families are notified of any change in status. Many programs offer follow-up care to facilities, as well. "Our program assists with transitions such as placement and other concerns once the discharge date has been decided," said Ms. Spadaro.

In my career I have witnessed the admittance of many individuals to this program. Like any other service, it is the family's responsibility to thoroughly investigate the program and seek references. However, a good gero-psych program may prove to be a very useful tool that can be successfully employed to help your loved one at this transitional time. If his behaviors are steadily worsening, you may need to seriously consider making an appointment with the director of a local program. This move may be the intervention necessary at this point in time. It also provides respite as you plan for home care or a move to a facility.

The following chapters will review the various care options available in order to prepare you to screen and choose the best possible quality of care and service for your loved one's needs.

10

HOME CARE SERVICES

A N INCREASINGLY POPULAR OPTION for families today is that of home care. Trained caregivers and companions may be retained to come to the home and provide services including:

- Laundry and light housekeeping
- Meal planning, preparation and shopping
- Medication reminders
- Transportation to medical appointments and errands
- Assistance with activities; interaction with client
- Observing, monitoring and reporting a client's condition

For those recovering from illness, personal care attendants and nurses aides can also perform the following services:

- Medication reminders
- Assistance with bathing, dressing and grooming
- Incontinence care
- Assistance with transfers and ambulating
- Monitoring food and fluid intake
- Monitoring and reporting skin conditions

Certified nurses' aides and home health aides for the critically ill or those needing intensive rehabilitation are qualified to carry out these additional duties:

- Emptying and caring for catheter or ostomy bag
- Assisting with exercises and rehabilitation activities
- Assistance with procedures as directed by the plan of care
- Identification and reporting of signs and symptoms needing attention

COSTS

Payment is private and is not covered by Medicare. Most services are structured to charge by the hour, with hourly rates ranging from $10 to $22. National averages indicate rates of $17 per hour for companions/homemakers and $19 for home health aides. The programs usually have a minimum number of hours per week. Services are available for day, evening and graveyard shifts. Families may also utilize this service if the parent is hospitalized or currently residing in a preferred assisted living facility, but wish to have extra companion services or one-on-one attention.

WHAT YOU NEED TO KNOW

- Caregivers must be bonded and fully insured with medical liability insurance.
- Caregivers must be fingerprinted and have criminal background clearance.
- Caregivers must have TB clearance and have passed a pre-employment physical.
- Caregivers must have proof of Worker's Compensation coverage.

SCREEN THE ORGANIZATION

Be sure to find out how long the company has been in business and ask for references. Are there physicians and case managers who refer to the agency regularly? Contact these professionals.

Ask to speak with the director or owner. Does he personally employ the caregiver? How does the company ensure that their caregivers provide excellent service? Who monitors the cases? How are potential problems identified and handled? What is their philosophy of service? What kind of additional background checks do they perform on their caregivers? Do they ensure that employees may legally work? Who is their most frequent source of referrals? Who owns the company? Does he have a medical or social services background? How is the company structured for accountability in the areas of taxes, Worker's Comp, and compliance with other legal requirements? Visit the organization's local office rather than simply retaining a caregiver by phone. Check for proper display of licenses and other professional credentials.

Inquire as to how the company promotes continuity of their work force. See if the organization offers health benefits, 401K or retirement plans. How do they recruit their staff? Do they have caregivers that have responsibly and successfully completed successive or long-term assignments?

CHOOSING THE RIGHT CAREGIVER

Inquire about the process of matching a caregiver to a client. How does the company determine who would be the best fit? What would be the deciding factor? Does the organization ever turn down cases? What happens if your parent takes a dislike to the caregiver? How are the caregivers trained? What educational or vocational preparation do they have for this job? Who in the agency supervises them? How are they equipped to handle special needs, such as dementia? How does the caregiver handle a difficult or confused client? Do certain caregivers have training for a specific diagnosis?

EXTRA CONSIDERATIONS

If English is the language spoken in your household, you need to make sure that the caregiver can communicate clearly in English. Does the caregiver know how to speak to someone who has a hearing or memory impairment without sounding condescending or overly loud? Does she demonstrate patience with the most frustrating behaviors? Is she flexible in allowing family input or does she resent it?

If your family member is of a particular ethnic or cultural persuasion, request a caregiver with the same background, especially if your parent converses in a native tongue or has always eaten foods that are not standard American fare. Clients who suffer from dementia sometimes experience paranoia and in some cases may view the caregiver as a threat. Chances are better in these cases that if the caregiver is from the same background she may appear less threatening. The goal is to make the transition as smooth as possible.

REPORTING

What is the reporting procedure? If a caregiver observes a change worth noting, how does she handle it? Is a supervisor notified? What if the family is unavailable? Who contacts the doctor? Do they have a network of healthcare specialists they recommend if needed? Are supervisors able to be reached on an on-call, "24/7" basis or would the employee reach a voice mail system after hours?

RECORD KEEPING

Most agencies will supply a logbook that serves to track time sheets, expenses, receipts and other details. If they do not, be sure to arrange with the caregiver a simple system by which she can log all pertinent expenditures and other information.

Make sure that the caregiver is supplied with necessary funds for groceries, medications, outings and basic supplies. Reconcile receipts regularly to avoid problems, and check them carefully. All purchases should reflect the needs of the senior; so make sure that the items on the grocery list are appropriate. Figure out in advance how much should be purchased, (or for best results order food online). Lead your caregiver not into temptation by limiting her access to cash, and by all means make sure that the checkbook is not accessible (you don't want the senior writing checks, either). All major household expenses should be handled separately and you want to ensure that this happens by having statements and bills mailed to your home. Do not give your parent large sums of cash – rather, dole it out weekly.

Have a separate logbook for visitors to sign if the immediate family lives out of area. This can be useful to screen and document any unwelcome visits.

TRANSPORTATION

Most agencies charge the family for use of the caregiver's vehicle if used to transport the senior. The usual fee is about .40 per mile and is added to the hourly rate. Reputable agencies check the employee's DMV records and verify insurance and registration on the caregiver's car. Be sure to make certain that the car is in good repair. Is it hard to get the client into the car? Watch to make sure that the caregiver can safely assist client into car. Are the seat belts functional? Are the tires in good shape? Does she have room to load a wheelchair or walker? How about a sliding board to help load a heavyset client? If vehicle is elevated, how can the client get in?

One option some agencies allow is to have the caregiver drive the client's car. In this situation it is the client's responsibility to insure, register and properly maintain the car. In these situations, mileage reimbursement is usually not applied.

ERROR-FREE ERRANDS

Ask the caregiver about running errands. She needs to carry a cell phone with emergency phone numbers. If she accompanies your parent to the market, she needs to make sure that your parent does not fiddle with stacked cans or step into a newly mopped area. (Only mildly confused seniors should go on banking or shopping errands). If the senior is seeing a new doctor or dentist, ensure that you or the caregiver calls in advance to let staff know that their patient has a cognitive impairment. They will appreciate your thoughtfulness and can assist the caregiver if she is called away momentarily (parking the car, etc). You don't want your loved one unsupervised even for a minute.

ESTABLISHING GOOD ROUTINES

If your loved one has energy to burn, he will need to have an outlet. Establish a regular exercise routine with the caregiver. Daily walks in the neighborhood should occur if there is no flight risk involved. Buy a plastic beach ball to toss back and forth. Most seniors have more energy in the morning, which is the best time for exercise. If your parent is afflicted with Sundowner's,** he will likely pace about in the evening, so exercise will need to be conducted at that time as well. Because you are dealing with limited attention spans, recognize that exercise periods may need to start and stop throughout the day. You'll need a caregiver that understands this and is flexible.

If your parent always enjoyed working in the yard, sweeping the porch or folding clothes, have the caregiver supervise these projects. Don't consider this real cleaning, as the job will usually be abandoned shortly. These tasks may be performed over and over and are good re-directional tools.

** Name of syndrome associated with dementia; refers to set of behaviors including suspicion, disorientation, heightened agitation, and restlessness and characterized by onset occurring at end of day/early evening.

"An effective caregiver will give her clients opportunities to promote their independence," asserts Rick Davis, president of Attentive Home Care in Orange, CA. "Racing to do everything for a client diminishes that person's sense of confidence that he is capable of doing for himself." Make sure your caregiver has the imagination and dedication to encourage the senior to maintain as much independence as he can.

SENSITIVITY COUNTS

If the senior has been moved to your home or a facility and he is mildly confused, do not allow visits to "go see" his former home. This is terribly upsetting to the individual and he may refuse to leave. I have seen well-meaning friends or caregivers take a resident out for a ride and visit to the old homestead, with disastrous results. This gesture can confuse and aggravate the senior and upset him greatly.

DINING

Discretion should always be used in regards to dining out. A quick salad at an informal fast-food joint is a fun outing for a mildly or moderately confused senior, but sit-down meals at a restaurant are usually out of the question. Short attention spans and shaky table manners make for an awkward dining experience and you do not want to prod or rush your loved one or have him stared at by others. Alert, well-trained caregivers should be regularly monitoring the client's weight gain or loss, in addition to keeping an eye on her eating habits and noting changes or problems with dietary intake.

Unless the caregiver is a registered dietician or chef, prepare meals yourself or write out meal plans and menus and have the ingredients easily accessible. You want to be sure that in your absence your loved one receives varied and square meals. The caregiver has neither the time nor the training to initiate meal planning. Remove the guesswork. Keep it simple and nutritious. Remember that your loved one may be confused but still likes and dislikes certain foods. Make clear any special needs that your parent has (food pureed or cut, allergic reactions, hatred of brussel sprouts, etc.) If your parent is in the latter stages of dementia, chewing will be increasingly difficult and you must guard against choking hazards. Eliminate stringy meats, popcorn or coarsely textured foods and stick with soft, easy-to-swallow staples. Your parent may dislike wearing dentures and complain that they hurt. Make some delicious, healthful smoothies or shakes. (You can add some boosters of protein in them.)

Food is often used as a diversionary tool for bored or agitated seniors, as long as it is healthy and the quantities are modest. Keep tasty, low-cal snacks on hand that the caregiver may use in those situations.

Sometimes a favorite food or treat can be used as rewards to coax clients who are struggling with certain tasks such as bathing or toileting. Apprehension or agitation that a senior might experience towards a difficult task or routine can be minimized, for instance, with the knowledge that he will eat chocolate ice cream afterwards.

Professional caregivers will appreciate your commitment to your relative. If a caregiver or agency is surprised by or resentful of your thoroughness, take your business elsewhere.

Once you've selected your caregiver, it is time to prepare for her arrival.

11

PUTTING YOUR HOUSE IN ORDER

SAFEGUARDING A HOME IN order to protect your loved one requires work and a willing spirit (especially if the house contains years of accumulated "goodies" and rooms rich in memorabilia but poor in organization). It is essential, however, to ensure that the confused individual resides in a home as free of potential hazards as possible.

PREPARATION FOR THE JOB:

If the house has more objects than floor space, you need to brace yourself and start de-junking. Fall risks and fire are two good reasons why you must restore order to the home. If the thought of sifting through mounds of old stuff staggers you, look in your handy directory. There are agencies that specialize with helping families downsize entire households. Rates for the services are reasonable and families often gladly divide the cost of the fee in exchange for allowing the heavy work to be done by outsiders. I recommend that you attack one room at a time by assessing which rooms are most infrequently used and then locking them until you are ready to work on them. This way you won't see chaos at every turn and lose heart.

If you are on a tight budget, try your local church or community center and see if they offer assistance.

Many cities have "Family Fix-It-Days" in which volunteers give up a Saturday and work on a senior citizen's house, performing tasks ranging from painting to cleaning and repair work. If you have a large family or circle of friends, prevail upon them. Have a work party and buy a couple of pizzas for your labor force.

Be sensitive to your loved one. Work should be performed when the senior is not around, in order to avoid unnecessary upset. Have the caregiver or a relative take mom out for the afternoon while you and the others get busy.

Let's take a look at the various areas of home and yard that will require your attention:

FURNISHINGS – Keep furniture and large items in the same spot, but free up as much floor space as possible. While your loved one may be confused, she likely knows her way around the house, and if she has any visual impairment, should not risk an accident that could happen if she sits down in a space that no longer contains her favorite chair.

While the location of the furnishings should remain the same, the pieces may be substituted if necessary.

Keep in mind that decreased mobility will be an issue to face in the near future. Could a wheelchair or walker be easily maneuvered in the house, or is there too little space? Is the sofa deep and hard to rise from? Is there an ottoman that protrudes and could be tripped over? If so, get rid of it. Replace the recliner chair (which can tip and is a hazard to manipulate) and substitute a solid straight-backed wing chair.

In some cases there may be rooms whose use should be discontinued. An example of this would be a sunken living room. Discourage the use of this room by darkening it and blocking it off. Move the television and easy chair into the den, bedroom or dining room and set up operation there. The senior will adapt.

Make sure that any large cabinets, hutches or grandfather clocks are securely bolted to the wall. Check the hallways and any rooms in use to ensure they are also free of objects that could be run into or tripped over. Watch for frayed carpeting and remove any heavy mirrors or wall hangings that could be grabbed if the senior lost his balance. Buy attractive wood moldings and install for use as handrails.

GARAGE – Does your parent own a car? Most seniors suffering from dementia think fondly of their car and still believe they are capable of driving. If your parent is in the early stages of dementia, he will likely mention the car and talk frequently of driving it. At this point it would be very traumatic to take the car away (later, the car will be forgotten). Disable the engine so that the car cannot run. Have the caregiver and your parent "visit" the car regularly as an activity. This can be very pleasing to males, who often will assert that they "need to go to" the car. A few moments sitting in the car is very pleasurable and will satisfy most people. If dad loved tinkering with the car, provide some wrenches and let him "teach" his caregiver about car repair. Eventually the car will be forgotten and can be disposed of.

While you are checking the garage, be sure to remove all solvents, old paint cans, sharp tools, and miscellany. You don't need your parent attempting to climb onto someone's old unicycle. The garage should be empty save for a workbench with a few benign tools and a broom. Any boxes stored should be fastened tightly with packing tape. Make sure that a padlock or automatic door system keeps the garage from being entered unexpectedly.

YARD – Make sure that the backyard is pleasant for sitting, as nature has a soothing effect on agitated persons and everyone needs regular exposure to sunshine. Purchase a hummingbird feeder for your parent's viewing enjoyment. Most home improvement stores sell moderately priced wall-mounted waterfalls. These provide diversions and relaxing sounds, without the danger of drowning. Pools or freestanding fountains should be drained or securely surrounded by locked fencing. Do NOT allow any caregiver to have access to the pool, even if she thinks a "dip" would be nice on a hot day. The senior should never be exposed to this potential hazard under any circumstances.

If your relative remembers a loving spouse, think about carving a big heart in a backyard tree with an inscription such as "Bill Loves Lila", their wedding date, or something sentimental. This provides a conversation point for the caregiver and is a lovely landmark for the family to enjoy.

Some seniors with dementia feel the need to be on the go. Many recall the days when they caught a bus to go to work or get around town. If this is the case, you will go a long way to helping accommodate this driving need if you construct a simple "bus stop" and erect it in the corner of your garden. Ask some teenage boys in your family to help assemble a makeshift stop. (I have had success with scout troops and local boys' and girls' clubs in obtaining their help for such projects).

Access to the front yard should be blocked. Make sure any garden gates connecting the two yards are sturdy and securely locked. Unless a high wall or gate encloses the front yard, you will need to be careful that the senior is not able to wander away. Encourage the caregiver to spend most time outside in the back yard.

Make sure that the front door has a good locking mechanism and a solid screen, preferably a one-way model which will allow air flow but guarantee greater privacy from outside eyes.

If the yard has a great deal of vegetation, hire a laborer and get all of that brush, ivy or excess growth cleaned out and the trees cut way back. You don't want your parent sticking his hand in a big bush and brushing up against a rat or animal unexpectedly. The undergrowth is always dusty and dirty and full of cobwebs, so get rid of it. Rose bushes and bougainvillea are lovely, but I recommend replacing all sharp, thorny plants in the house or yard with low-maintenance flowering plants. If you do not plan to retain a gardener or foresee yourself working in the yard, clear out these plants and replace them with bark or stone. Make sure that there are no poisonous plants in the house or yard that could be ingested (poinsettia, oleander, etc.)

Throw out cracked pots and make sure there are no old rusty tools or sharp discarded gardening implements from decades ago. If there is a shed, make sure it is locked at all times and the key out of reach.

See if there are any missing bricks or uneven paving that could trigger a tumble. Have a gardener lower any raised sprinkler heads to below lawn level.

Place a sturdy glider chair under a tree for afternoon siestas. If yard is sun-drenched, purchase an umbrella/chair arrangement for relief from the hot rays (or the caregiver will never use the yard).

Check to make sure wall or fence dividing property from the neighbors does not have missing pieces or "escape hatches."

KITCHEN – Clean out the refrigerator and cupboards, removing old foods that have outlasted their expiration date. Remove any foods that are inappropriate if your parent has special dietary restrictions (sugary items for a diabetic, etc.).

Buy attractive, dishwasher-safe, plastic dinnerware. Because those with dementia often struggle with depth perception, they need brightly colored plates with divided sections in order to distinguish foods. As dementia advances, it often attacks motor skills and if a senior cannot feed himself, he will stop trying. Place one fork next to the plate (don't confuse the person with multiple silverware). Pour liquids into a pretty sipper-style cup if grasping a regular glass is too difficult and causes spills. Most stores carry good-looking vinyl place mats and tablecloths that are durable and easy to wipe.

Work with the caregiver to develop ways in which the senior can keep busy during meal preparation. The goal is to keep the person away from a hot stove. Suggest that the food be cooked during a rest or nap period. Perhaps you can assign the senior a task such as table setting or napkin folding. Give the person a very simple job that he can complete or attempt with little frustration. Keep all knives out of reach, and remind the caregiver that meals should take only a few minutes to prepare because the senior needs constant monitoring.

If the senior is shaky, utilize a good-looking cummerbund-style bib to protect his clothing during mealtimes. (See Chapter 21)

RECREATION AREA – Have a designated area set aside for physical activity. If you have a loved one with energy to burn, set out a supply of exercise videos, music tapes and CD's (for dancing). Thrift stores usually have an abundance of tapes to choose from for less than a dollar. Make sure that you have a caregiver who is peppy and willing to "work out" with your parent. Your parent needs regular exercise, not just for the enjoyment and diversion of a fun activity, but to preserve muscle tone and strength.

PETS – If there is a furry friend in the house, makes sure that you or the caregiver is supervising the feedings and that the animal is not overfed or neglected. Do not keep a pet that could scratch or turn on the senior if the person becomes agitated. If the creature is docile and your loved one still enjoys holding and petting it, then by all means, keep Fluffy. You will need to take into account the needs of the pet when interviewing caregivers. Some may be allergic to or afraid of animals and you will need to see if they will require additional fees for cleaning up and caring after the pet.

Anticipate the unforeseen and you won't be caught unprepared.

CLEANING – If house has been dirty and dusty for some time, professionally clean upholstery, drapes and carpeting. If possible, replace these items. Consider purchasing a quality air filter, which will help rid the house of dander, dust and pollen.

Check for bug infestation, which often occurs if the senior has been hoarding food or excessive numbers of stray animals. If the parent has neglected the home for some time, there may be a termite problem to address.

Give away or discard as much clutter as possible. No one will miss it.

OTHER DOORS – Make sure any basement or attic doors are locked. Put child-resistant locks on all cabinet doors. Install a peephole on the front door – your caregiver will thank you. Make sure that the front door has multiple locks, as a senior in the early stages of dementia may still be capable of opening a simple bolt-type arrangement.

BEDROOM – Check to see that there is no heavy shelf or hanging object over or near the bed. The bedroom needs a night light, but place it out of sight so it does not annoy your loved one and risk its being touched or "fixed." Make sure that your linen closet has bedding for cool and warm weather and remind the caregiver that these need to be changed out at the turning of the seasons. Reduce all clutter to a minimum. Store or get rid of breakable knickknacks and fragile figurines. Display photo albums and photographs that may be discussed and looked at as an activity.

Seniors who experience paranoia or delusional behavior can become easily frightened by reflected images. If you see this happening, remove or drape the dresser mirror and any others. Keep colors soft and soothing – avoid loud bedspreads and designs. Eliminate the danger of falling objects by replacing hanging pictures with pretty borders or simple hand-painted sponge patterns.

If your loved one has a room with a street view, relocate him to a back bedroom (if there is another with an attached or nearby bath). If not, replace the curtains with blinds or shutters in front of the window.

Female caregivers will particularly appreciate this gesture, especially in the evenings. You don't need outsiders watching intimate routines.

Blocking your windows will also discourage the senior from peeking out, as the blinds will be too confusing to operate. Another suggestion is to purchase one of those "view" inserts that fit into a window frame and create instant seascapes or mountain panoramas.

Large picture windows need to have a chair or some sizeable item blocking them, if possible, lest a confused person risks walking through a clean, transparent one by accident. Consider installing inexpensive blinds, or if the house is dark and needs sunlight, put a sofa in front of the living room window. You can buy inexpensive decals to paste onto the glass to aid in this effort.

CLOSETS – Weed out closets and drawers. Throw out all shoes with dangerous or worn heels. Replace skimpy, often-washed nightwear with modest pajamas or nightgowns. Your parent does not need an overstuffed closet full of outdated clothing. She needs attractive, functional garments that can be interchanged and easily donned. The outfits also need to be made of durable material that can withstand regular washing. Be thoughtful and don't buy mom form-fitting white pants if she wears briefs that would be visible or bulky. A simple cotton skirt would be more flattering and dignified.

Check for hidden money in old purses or boxes. Frightened seniors will often hoard money, jewelry or food if they believe they are being watched. Check all pockets, socks, and bags that you may find stuffed in a drawer or closet. Purchase a few wallets or purses (as they will disappear), and put some change and a dollar or two in the billfold. Add to a lady's purse some tissue, hair combs and a light lipstick. These are good re-directional tools and provide the senior pleasure, as well as some harmless items to fiddle with.

While cleaning out closets, make a point of checking all cabinets for dangerous solvents, alcohol, and even nail polish. Scissors, tweezers and sharp instruments should be out of reach as well. You must assume that your parent has the discretion of a tiny child. When in doubt, put the item up high.

Sift carefully through drawers as you may find important papers stuck in odd places. Set aside any heirlooms in a special box and arrange with your siblings to safely store expensive jewelry or valuable items in a safety-deposit box. Assemble any official documents, files and sensitive information and arrange to take it home. (You don't want an agitated parent destroying crucial paperwork or risk having this confidential information falling into the wrong hands). Do make sure, though, that the caregiver has your parent's medical card, emergency phone numbers and information prominently located near the phone. Have an extra copy made listing current medications and other pertinent medical information, place in a clear plastic sheet protector and tape it out of reach on the inside of your front door. This will aid paramedics greatly in the event that they are summoned to the house.

For added protection, contact the Alzheimer's Association for information on obtaining a "Safe Return" bracelet in the event that your parent wanders from the home.

BATHROOM – Make sure that the toilet is easily accessible. If the bathroom adjoining the bedroom is tiny, remove the connecting door from the hinges to allow for more maneuverability. Make sure that shampoos, lotions and grooming toiletries are safely locked up.

Check the medicine cabinet for old medications and destroy them.

Install grab bars near the toilet and also in the shower. Purchase a shower chair and attach a hand-held nozzle for easy use by the caregiver. Discourage the caregiver from using the tub as it is too difficult to help the senior in and out safely and easily. Use the shower instead. If the home has only bathtubs, contract with a local company that specializes in cutting down the bathtub walls for easy step-in. (Most companies charge about $400 to do the job). Make sure that the tub has a slip-proof pad and rugs near the tub, toilet and sink.

STAIRS – If there is a stairway, set up the downstairs to accommodate all of the senior's needs. Your loved one should not be using the stairway under any circumstances. If the caregiver consistently redirects and utilizes the first floor areas, the senior will forget about the existence of the upper floor.

Block off the stairs as best as you can. If you live on the second floor, you will need to experiment with ways that you can get upstairs with minimal hassle, and don't let the senior see you ascend. Attach some fabric to a rope and cordon off the area. Stick a large fern in front of it and you'll still be able to get upstairs with little difficulty, while preventing your parent from climbing up. If your loved one is still fairly coherent, he may ask. Simply respond to questions by stating that you "can't go up because the floors are wet," and redirect him. Soon he will cease to care about or notice the stairway.

APPLIANCES – Ensure that irons and other appliances are stored and out of reach. Block electrical outlets and cap off any not in use. Cover the top of your stove when not in use (you can buy burner covers). Make sure no wires are exposed and those cords are not frayed. If your parent has a house full of antiques, check every lamp. If your parent is tempted to change light bulbs, remove the lamp and put in track lighting or mount a light fixture high on the ceiling, out of reach. Electrocution is a very real hazard and must be guarded against at all costs. Instruct the caregiver to keep curling irons and hair dryers out of sight and replace old appliances (coffee makers, irons) with newer models that include an automatic-shut off system. Make sure night-lights are in every room and all hallways.

Avoid stacking items. Recently, the news reported a tragic death involving a little boy that climbed on a dresser in an attempt to pull down a huge television set. The child was crushed in the process. Don't let this happen to your loved one. Walk through each room with a critical eye and imagine scenarios that a curious or frustrated person might create.

Start your relationship off right by asking your caregiver for her thoughts, as she has likely helped other families safeguard their homes, too.

12

RESPITE STAYS

RESPITE STAYS HAVE BECOME increasingly popular in the last ten years. This short-term alternative or precursor to permanent placement allows a tired caregiver a period of rest while his loved one is in the care of others at a facility.

Most communities charge fees ranging from $70 to $200 per day for a respite stay, and many places have a minimum required stay of one week to 30 days. Respite stays assist the families by providing an opportunity for families who wish to travel, take care of pressing business (surgery, home sale, moving/relocation, wedding) and also may be utilized to help families begin to consider a more permanent arrangement outside of the home. For some, a respite stay simply provides a much-needed break from the rigors of caring for an afflicted individual.

I have often recommended respite visits as a "trial stay" for families who are largely convinced that it is time for a move, but who were still guilt-ridden about committing to it. Some families' find that a respite stay is offers the perfect chance to begin the emotional adjustment that is needed when handing over care of their parent to outsiders.

Some families need to ensure that the move to a facility is the best decision, as they worry that their loved one will not have a positive experience. A respite stay allows the family to witness the senior adapting (in most cases) fairly easily to a new routine, provided he is receiving attentive and consistent care.

ARRANGING A RESPITE STAY

Using the aforementioned resource guides, contact the appropriate local facilities and ask for information on respite visits. Most licensed facilities do offer this program; they will usually jump at the chance to coordinate a respite stay (in the hopes that you will be convinced that the facility can meet your loved one's needs and consider a permanent arrangement). Short-term stays are usually simple to arrange and admittance to the program will be granted provided:

- **There is a bed available** (some facilities have a designated private, furnished respite room while others may simply offer an empty bed in a shared unit).
- **The client passes** TB clearance. Do NOT consider any facility that would waive this requirement.
- **A physician's report** is completed and signed by examining medical doctor.
- The **responsible party reviews and signs** all paperwork (necessary even for a short-term respite stay).
- The **family pays** in advance for all services.
- The **client meets** assessment criteria.
- The **family commits** to a designated minimum stay (will range from one week to one month, usually. Most facilities discourage shorter stays due to the amount of paperwork, staffing and transition involved).

Most facilities hope that a respite stay will be the "icing on the cake" which will convince the family that the client can be well served in this setting, and that the next step to take following a successful respite is a permanent move. In most cases the transition is a fairly simple and seamless one, as *both* the client and the family have already begun to acclimate.

13

ADULT DAY PROGRAMS

ONE VIABLE OPTION FOR families to consider is to enroll their relative in an adult day care program. Most communities have centers that offer this service to the public. Some are sponsored by hospitals, non-profit organizations or various private agencies run others. These programs may be located on the grounds of a senior center, hospital, church, office building, or other setting. Centers are open usually five days a week, excluding holidays and weekends.

HOW IT WORKS

There are two types of programs that a center can facilitate. These are classified as **adult day health care** (medical model) and **adult day care** (social model) programs. You will need to decide which program your loved one needs.

Adult day health care refers to a program that offers monitoring of medical conditions under the supervision of a medical director. A registered nurse and nurses' aides assist participants in the program. These professionals, along with a Master's level social worker and activity leader, are mandated to provide physical care. Medication can be administered, blood pressure and blood sugar checks are performed, and rest areas are provided for the client. Families are reassured to know that their loved one will have an opportunity to join in thoughtfully planned activities without his physical needs being overlooked.

Seniors with dementia not requiring the same degree of medical monitoring utilize **adult day care** programs – which simply means that the day's activities are designed for clientele who do not require the same degree of medical attention. Because the clients are generally in good health, the daily calendar of activities in this type of program resemble those of a senior center more than that of a nursing facility.

Facilities that offer both programs all have their own format. Some integrate their clients, while others offer a program within a program – meaning that those with greater medical needs have separate activities from the other population.

Most facilities are licensed as adult day health centers. To qualify for this program, an assessment is necessary. The RN, in conjunction with the social worker and other staff determine eligibility and develop a comprehensive care plan for the senior. The objective is to identify the problem in context of what determines intervention and then formulate an appropriate plan of action. The multi-disciplinary team confers to review the social and/or health needs of the applicant.

SAFETY FIRST

Safety of the participant is a key factor in determining eligibility in most programs. The facilities offer some degree of security, including alarms on doors and a delayed egress system (which has to do with slowed timing of doors being opened as a result of being pushed or leaned on). Some programs are better equipped to facilitate serious flight risks as they are designed with special secured areas for clients who tend to wander.

Families who face this challenge should inquire on tour about this. In facilities that do not offer secured sections the staff can redirect mild wanderers, but are usually unable to handle those insistent upon leaving the program.

STAFFING

Staffing is based on attendance levels. Because the state requires a high ratio of staff to participant, the attendees receive considerable supervision. Due to the nature of the service provided, it is mandatory for the facility to retain licensed professionals on staff. Because virtually all administrative and line staff also interact with the participants, they are usually well trained and adept at dealing with the behavioral challenges a senior may present.

COSTS

These programs average about $76 (Medi-Cal reimbursement rate) per day for adult day health care. The Center is required to charge the same amount as Medi-Cal reimburses, and fees for the medical model are based according to a *daily* rate. Those requiring the services of this program have medical needs that demand constant oversight. Because of this, many participants are eligible for funding assistance. In California those who qualify receive funding for an average two days of the program. (Each state varies in terms of funding offered, and with budget cuts occurring in many parts of the country there is no way to determine what will be available from year to year.)

According to Susan Lawton, M.S.W., director of A Day Away Adult Day Health Care Center, approximately 95% of participants in adult day health care programs statewide are currently receiving Medi-Cal benefits. For those beginning the process, the first step would be for the facility to submit a doctor's statement outlining the need for placement in the program.

OTHER FUNDING SOURCES

Some long-term insurance policies, along with health care policies, such as SCAN, may pay for adult day health care services. The Veteran's Administration has agreements with individual contract-authorized providers as well.

For those paying privately costs average about $69 a day for adult day health care. Adult day care that does not involve health monitoring charges by the *hour* at a rate of about $7 an hour, with meals included. Medi-Cal, Medicare or most insurance plans do not cover social model programs. Facilities typically require a commitment of at least several hours a day or several days a week.

ACTIVITIES

Activities are integrated, and participants who have experienced social isolation or trouble relating to a caregiver often respond well to the program. Periodic reviews analyze not only any health issues but also the socialization progress of a participant.

Susan Lawton emphasizes that many studies have borne out the fact that effective socialization is as crucial a factor in aging well as is diet and exercise. She adds that the biggest challenge adult day centers face "is making families aware of the many benefits of the program for both the senior and the caregiver."

TOURING

Touring the center and reviewing the adult day programs is not as time-consuming as investigating a residential live-in care facility. Arrange to have a tour and meeting with the program director and block about one to two hours to ensure adequate time to view the facility, meet the staff, and become thoroughly acquainted with the program.

These programs have helped many seniors enjoy a more varied, stimulating daily routine while providing a needed respite for the caregiver. Families who are also considering an eventual move to a residential facility have benefited from these day programs as they learn to "let go" and allow their loved one to receive assistance from other care providers.

14

CHOOSING A FACILITY

WHEN THE FAMILY AND physician have reached an agreement that it is no longer feasible to keep the senior at home, the appropriate facility needs to be carefully selected. Decision-makers often hesitate, understandably, at initiating the next step, paralyzed by the possibilities lurking in their minds:

- Fear of choosing the wrong facility
- Fear that the senior will be traumatized by the move
- Worry that their loved one would not adapt to the environment
- Fear that the wrong move would add more financial stress and be more costly
- Fear that upheaval would be too difficult for the senior
- Fear of losing control over.care of their loved one
- Fear of abuse, theft
- Fear that botched move would result in an even more difficult transition

These are legitimate concerns that any caring, conscientious care provider may have. In this chapter we will differentiate between the various types of care facilities, highlight their services and outline steps that you can take to ensure that the senior is appropriately placed and is receiving quality care.

A WORD ON LICENSING STANDARDS

All licensed care facilities are regulated by the Department of Social Services and must meet certain criteria specific to the type of care that they offer. This may seem like an obvious fact with large, institutional settings, but small residential board and care homes are also beholden to the same licensing standards.

Never consider moving your loved one to any unlicensed setting.

Regulatory practices and standards vary from state to state. Later in this chapter you will find a list of questions that you need to have answered by the administrator of the facility that you are considering for your loved one. One important question will deal with how the facility performed on the comprehensive survey that the Department of Social Services' Community Care licensing division conducts over a period of 1-2 days at the site on an annual or semi-annual basis. This survey reviews every operating aspect of the institution – from investigating the physical plant and its maintenance, to reviewing files and record keeping. Poor scores result in citations and possible fines. You will need to find out the survey results of any facility you are seriously looking into. The facility will have a record and you can contact the DSS office in your area to ask who their liaison is for that particular facility.

WHAT TYPE OF FACILITY IS BEST?

If it has been determined that a parent is no longer capable of residing at home and living with family is not an option, the choice of an appropriate facility opens up several possibilities. We will look at the options available.

At this time, there are an abundance keep of centers equipped to offer dementia care, but how do you know which would be best? When evaluating, keep in mind the following:

- Physical/medical needs
- Degree of cognitive impairment
- Proximity to your home
- Type of resident population
- Affordability
- Philosophy of care
- Your "gut instinct"

SKILLED NURSING, ASSISTED LIVING, & BOARD AND CARE HOMES

Generally speaking, there are three types of care facilities that you will need to distinguish from in order to begin to determine which would best suit the needs of your loved one. These are:

- SKILLED NURSING FACILITIES
- ASSISTED LIVING FACILITIES
- BOARD AND CARE HOMES

Each type of facility offers dementia care. Step one requires determining the physical needs of the senior, as he must meet certain medical criteria that distinguish one institution from another. Skilled nursing facilities offer a greater degree of medical services, while the latter two are considered a "social model" in terms of structure. First we will differentiate between the medical services each type of facility offers.

SKILLED NURSING FACILITIES (commonly referred to as "nursing homes" or "SNF's") offer medical care and monitoring to patients with acute physical needs. Your parent is best suited for a skilled nursing facility if his needs meet the following criteria:
- Bed-bound
- Requires intravenous feedings
- Requires care for advanced wounds (designated by stages)
- Non-ambulatory, non weight-bearing
- Unable to feed self
- Uses liquid oxygen
- Requires frequent insulin injections and shots[***]
- Has permanent indwelling catheter[****]

Skilled nursing facilities benefit patients with these needs:
- Ongoing acute physical care and monitoring of conditions
- Daily access to medical professionals
- Protection from falls

Not all SNF's offer dementia care, but some do. Some facilities will take patients who suffer from mild dementia as long as they do not pose a flight risk. This is usually because the facility does not have a separate, secured area in the building. This is not recommended unless the patient is staying for a short-term visit, as the staff likely does not have much training in how to facilitate the non-medical needs of the confused patient. Look for a SNF that can handle both.

■ *Daily Routine*
Patients who are able are usually up early and wheeled or escorted to a main dining area for a meal. Activity directors, volunteers or adult education teachers interact with the patients

---

[***] Some assisted living facilities retain visiting nurses who can administer injections to residents within certain guidelines

[****] Criteria for admission may vary in different states

and offer simple games, exercises and other stimulation. Most retire to their rooms shortly after dinner, which is served in the early evening.

■ *Challenges*

Families need to observe the level of activity offered and ensure that their loved one receives meaningful stimulation on a daily basis. This means checking to make sure that the patient is escorted to all activities and verifying events take place as scheduled.

Skilled nursing homes care for many ill patients. They face a constant challenge to keep the building clean and smelling fresh. This is not an impossible goal, and I have visited superb facilities that were dedicated to airing and scouring the building on a daily basis (note – this can be accomplished without overwhelming the inhabitants with the smell of ammonia!) You will need to observe the housekeeping and maintenance practices of the facility to determine whether or not cleanliness is a top priority.

If your parent is unable to leave her bed, you need to check to see the efficiency of the food distribution system. When I was volunteering at a SNF in college, I was dismayed to see how slow and ineffective that facility's system was in delivering meals to the bed-bound. Worse, the kitchen supervisor showed little concern when I pointed out that food was arriving late and cold to the hungry patients. I can still see her disinterested face 20 years later. Mistakes are forgivable, but you don't want your parent living where there is little regard given to the comfort and care of a patient.

If the facility is not housing your parent in a secured dementia unit, you will need to meet with the day, evening and overnight staff to make sure that they understand basic communication skills necessary in order to help a confused person who may be in distress. Make sure they are educated about dementia and its facets.

■ *Staffing*

Skilled nursing homes are staffed with RNs', social workers, licensed vocational nurses and certified nurses' aides. A director of nurses oversees the medical program, sometimes under the supervision of a physician, who is employed as medical director. A licensed administrator manages skilled nursing facilities. Other professionals working in tandem with the facility include physicians, psychiatrists, physical and occupational therapists, to name a few.

■ *Costs and Payment Information*

Skilled nursing fees for private and shared rooms are charged on a monthly basis, calculated at a daily rate. Rates vary greatly depending upon geographical location (compare Alaska's private rates of $570 per day for private accommodations to Louisiana's rate of $111). In California, families typically will find rates averaging from $70 to $200 per day. The 2006 Metropolitan Life Market Survey of Nursing Home and Home Care costs shows findings of a national average of $206 per day ($75,190 yearly) for private rooms and $183 ($66,795) for semi-private accommodations.

SNF's accept Medicare reimbursement, Medicaid (MediCal in California), some long-term health insurance policies, VA benefits and private pay as payment for services.

ASSISTED LIVING FACILITIES – These residential care facilities (commonly referred to as "retirement homes") house anywhere from 25 to several hundred residents in one congregate setting. Residents who do not need the medical services of a SNF benefit from the social stimulation and peer interaction that these communities offer. These facilities are good for residents who are in the early to mid stages of dementia and are fairly ambulatory or able to get around in a wheelchair. Ample grounds help those who have nervous energy or wander, since they are able to roam about.

As a larger community is usually more bustling, those who need to be amidst activity benefit from this environment.

■ *Daily Routine*

Residents are usually up at 7:00 a.m., bathed, dressed and in the communal dining and activity areas for the remainder of the day. Volunteers, teachers and activity directors will organize various classes, sing-a-longs, and other activities. Residents may be transported to medical appointments, but more frequently are treated at the facility by visiting nurses, doctors, and therapists.

■ *Challenges*

Due to the size of the resident population, it is more difficult for a resident to receive one-on-one attention. Some families may wish to accommodate this need by contracting with a home health companion to visit the resident for several hours each day or week.

Larger facilities may seem a bit overwhelming to the more reclusive or shy types. Families need to work with the staff in setting up a "buddy system" and other aids to help a resident who may find the first few weeks daunting.

Because assisted living facilities are not medical models, you will need to clarify how much training the staff has in anticipating changes in condition and physical infirmities. Many now hire nurses or nurses' aides to join their staff. Check the credentials of the staff and determine with whom they are aligned in the medical community. They should have good working relationships with reputable medical professionals, including an excellent hospice provider in the event that the resident requires these valuable services.

■ *Staffing*

Assisted living facilities are managed by an executive director and employ a director of resident care to oversee the program. Caregivers are trained according to guidelines set forth by the company and in compliance with licensing standards. Many companies hire nurses aides for these positions, and occasionally the directors of the property are nurses or former social workers. They are, however, limited in the types of medical services that they are allowed to perform, as the community's licensing restrictions apply to all staff, regardless of the individuals' credentials.

■ *Costs and Payment Information*

Rates vary greatly from place to place and are affected by many factors, including geography, age of the building, and other variables. Most fees are calculated by the day. Most communities opt to charge families base rent, and then add on care fees and miscellaneous costs, averaging several thousand dollars per month (See Chapter 15 for more details on costs of assisted living).

Assisted living communities accept long-term health insurance and special veterans' benefits, as well as private pay for treatment. Medicare is not accepted, as medical services are not provided.

BOARD AND CARE HOMES[*****] These are licensed small residential facilities, usually offering six to fourteen beds. These best serve individuals who do not require skilled nursing but who have special physical needs, particularly those considered fall risks. This is because the area is smaller than its assisted living counterparts, offering carpeted floors, and without elevators, stairs

---

[*****] Board and care homes may classify themselves as "assisted living", as they are licensed to offer those services. They are thus regulated by the same dictates of the DSS. For clarity, I have distinguished the two facilities by describing those institutions that facilitate more than 15 people as assisted living facilities and the smaller communities as board and care homes.

or other hazards. Shy, retiring non-social types often prefer these quieter environments. Frail residents with fairly acute dementia do well in these more sedentary environments, as they are usually beyond participating in many activities.

Advantages include easy access to management, as the owner is often the manager. Protocol is less formal in these smaller facilities, which may work well for a senior who has special demands. Family may also be able to enjoy greater flexibility in negotiating fees and any discounts that the owner may offer. Seniors who prefer a "homey" environment would find the transition easier, as well.

■ *Daily Routine*

Daily routine is very similar to that of a larger assisted living facility. The majority of activity occurs during the morning and afternoon, as that is when the resident has the highest levels of energy. Dinner is usually served in the late afternoon, followed by an early bedtime.

Some board and care facilities arrange for outside entertainers or teachers to conduct an activity or two at the home. Most rely upon the day staff to organize and carry out activities.

■ *Challenges*

Families need to evaluate the amount of stimulation available for their loved one. If the person is in an advanced stage of dementia, he will not require as much activity but still needs exercise and some degree of stimulation, other than television watching.

Meal preparation may be less sophisticated and varied. Check to see if there is a printed menu and if the staff adheres to it or just throws together a simple meal.

Smaller, more intimate environments may mean fewer professional standards of conduct. Staff needs to be attired properly and trained in correct dementia care. Make sure that English is clearly spoken and that all staff has clearance to work there. (I once performed an impromptu drop-in to check out a local board and care and was upset to find a school-age boy in attendance, cooking dinner. No adult was in sight).

■ Costs and Payment Information

Board and care homes operate on a private pay basis, with rates competitive to those of the larger assisted living facilities.

Subsequent chapters will address some of these issues and give you guidelines that you can follow when you visit the facilities and meet with the management. These will reinforce to you what you need to be aware of in any facility and how you can put the directors on alert that you are carefully monitoring the care of your loved one.

15

ARRANGING TO TOUR A FACILITY

TOURING IS THE FUN part – really! It's an eye opener (in some cases, a veritable eye-popper!), but it needn't be difficult, lengthy or taxing. You don't need to visit every place under the sun, and you can easily weed out the good places from the not-so-hot if you do a little homework in advance and know what to ask and look for.

Most families now visit a facility with some knowledge of what to inquire about. They may have been coached by a friend or have gotten some how-to's from a book or the Internet. This chapter will explore the pre-tour process including searching for a facility, making the preliminary phone call, and setting a tour.

These guidelines will vary a bit depending upon whether you are visiting a skilled nursing facility, residential board and care, or assisted living community, but overall you will find that they are applicable regardless of the type of service provided.

QUESTIONS MOST FAMILIES USUALLY ASK

- How much does this cost?
- How big are the rooms?
- How is the food?
- What if we have to move her out?
- What type of daily routine is there?

Families that experienced a satisfying tour and like the answers they received may strongly consider making a move. However, they have done little to ensure that they will get what they really need, which means superb, proactive care. Why? There are two reasons:

Families usually don't feel qualified in any way to monitor care and therefore feel uncomfortable discussing it

Families lack any sort of realistic yardstick by which to measure the services.

QUESTIONS FAMILIES NEED TO ASK

- Is the facility truly equipped to serve my loved one?
- How can I reduce the chances of making a bad placement?
- How can I determine that this is the best move for my loved one?
- How can I distinguish between "fluff" and the real thing?
- How do I avoid "buyer's remorse" and any unexpected surprises?

Remember, you are the potential paying customer and you have every right to ask detailed questions. Skillful marketing directors who are a proud part of a reputable facility are willing to share the facility's attributes with you and it is easy to verify if these practices occur as promised. Superior staff will not only be able to offer you a fine program but educate you as well if you came in looking for attractive craft rooms but don't realize you should be more interested in how the medications room is organized. Your liaison should serve as teacher, not a guide in a showroom.

PRE-TOUR CONSIDERATIONS

When shopping for a facility, it is best to start by taking into consideration:

- **Location**
- **Price**
- **Nature of services**

Location

Most families want to be in close proximity to the facility, so factor in traffic time if you intend to visit the facility frequently. Don't rule out, though, facilities that are a little farther away if the care is exceptional. The more needy the senior, however, the closer your selection should be as you will want to be able to run over in the event of a problem.

If the caregiver is looking into making a move to a retirement community simultaneously or soon thereafter, shop for a facility that offers a dementia wing or look for one that is located within an easy driving distance. Some communities will even coordinate transportation for the well spouse to go and visit the senior.

You'll need to know if the neighborhood is generally safe. Is it in a residential or business area? Residential is preferable in the event that the senior wanders away (can't get onto a busy highway quickly. If you are seriously considering a quality facility located on a busy street, double check the security system. See if they take group walks in the neighborhood or if they drive residents to a park or safer area in which to have a constitutional.

Location may also determine the stability of the employee pool. I once worked in a beautiful, five-star community in an affluent hilltop neighborhood. Because service professions don't pay much, it was hard to attract staff to clean, wash and give care. The well-to-do housewives and teenagers in the area did not need to make extra money with a part-time job. There was also no bus stop in the area, so we couldn't draw employees from other locales. The developers were counting on the lovely view to be the selling point. They were right – for about the first two minutes on tour. There was a constant shortage of employees.

Older neighborhoods can have dignity; so if you find out that a place you like is in an older part of town, don't reject the idea. Some facilities that offer great care at moderate rates can offer these reasonable fees because they have lower overhead. Drive by at night and see how well the community is illuminated. Check with your police department to see if there are many break-ins or vandalism in the area (you don't need your car constantly broken into). If you get a good report, by all means, consider the facility if they meet the other criteria.

Pricing

Pricing ranges according to region and state, and as with the housing market they will be impacted by geography and population. Desert or rural communities generally have lower rates than metropolitan or coastal locations. Make sure that you get a price breakdown in writing, with all fees listed.

There are excellent facilities in every price range, although it is difficult to find many that offer rates in the low-priced range (in Southern California, this would be under $1000 for assisted living and below $2000 for skilled nursing care). Operating costs, worker's comp, and other factors have driven up the costs. I agree that there is truth in the saying that you get what you pay for, but this does not mean that all lower or moderately priced programs are bad and that the pricier ones are better. Low-priced programs are fine if they prune the budget in the areas of entertainment, landscaping and fancy foods. It's okay if the carpet is old as long as it is clean, safe, and not threadbare. There's nothing wrong with a simple activity program, as long as it is varied and stimulating. Beautifully appointed, costly facilities don't mean much if they lack good, consistent care programs.

BREAKDOWN OF RATES IN ASSISTED LIVING & BOARD AND CARE HOMES

Rates are usually structured by factoring in three components – base rent, levels of care, and additional fees.

■ *Base rent* (includes room, meals, activities, laundry, and scheduled transportation). In 2007, averages in Southern California for base rent ranges from $800 to $4000.

■ *Levels of care* can range from two or three to about eight, but essentially offer the same services, including bathing, medication management, escorts to meals, and incontinence/toileting care. Lowest level of care is the least expensive because it requires minimal supervision. Prices here usually start around $400 and can run as high as $4000 for highest levels of care.

Ask about hidden fees, such as frequent transportation to doctor, incontinence supplies (not just garments, but wipes, gloves for staff, etc.), special laundry services for excessive wetters, and additional supervision for hard-to-manage types (wanderers, agitated types).

■ *Community fees* are separate, one-time sign-up charges, essentially. These can range from $300 to $7000 at the time of move-in. This fee is usually non-refundable and is like a fancy security deposit, although you don't get it back unless there is a sudden death or health decline in the first month of residency. Communities describe this as an administrative processing fee and will often negotiate this rate if a family member balks but is valued as a potential client.

Some communities roll all of the care into one fee, including the base rent. At any rate, the totals will usually be close. Communities are very competitive and you will not find wildly divergent rates within the industry (excepting very high-end or low-income facilities).

Show Me The Money

Receptionists in most communities are trained not to give out rates over the telephone. Sometimes they honestly don't know the prices, but you need to find out what the rates are before you spend any more time investigating. (There's no point in falling in love with a place that is way out of your price range). Most staffs are trained to hedge around the rate question because the company wants you to visit the facility before rates are divulged. Usually at this point in the call you will be put through to the marketing director. These professionals, too, are often directed not to reveal pricing. Politely inform the person that you need a ballpark number to see if this remotely works with your budget before either of you invest any more time. Seasoned professionals will tell you the rates because they have a more realistic understanding of the sales process.

Facilities often withhold rates until tour time because they legitimately believe that the family needs to understand why they are paying thousands of dollars a month. They know that the price can seem overwhelming when quoted over the phone. A good marketing director can quote rates but also pique enough curiosity to inspire the family to arrange a tour.

It is important to expect unforeseen costs and anticipate that you will end up paying more than originally planned for, as the disease is progressive.

Board and care homes also structure rates similarly, either with one all-inclusive total or several levels of services. Rates will be comparable to those of assisted living facilities. Community fees may be charged at the discretion of the proprietor, and can often be negotiated.

Payment for these types of programs is private. Long-term health care insurance and some veteran's benefits may apply. Skilled nursing facilities' prices range from $2000 on up and the social worker on staff can advise as to the amount of Medicare or other federal or state aid that is available.

Nature of Services

You will need to determine if this is a program specifically for dementia or if those with dementia are merely accommodated (some places have a dementia waiver but no real program). Some facilities have a separate unit or section for dementia, while most communities serve only that population. If the former is the case, then you will need to make certain that this is not an afterthought, but rather an independent, well-thought out program with specific care, training and activities geared toward their clients. Otherwise, you may get a community that has simply licensed a section of the building to accommodate additional residents, without a very specialized program. Check thoroughly. You want caregivers who work only in that section and who understand the needs of their charges. (Employees who float back and forth are usually not trained to handle dementia-related behaviors and may not feel comfortable or skilled in helping this population.)

PRELIMINARY PHONE CALL

Use your preliminary phone call to determine the tone of the facility. Does the receptionist sound disinterested or enthusiastic? Remember, front desk employees have key positions. They usually monitor the security system and have a close relationship with families, summon paramedics in emergencies and help coordinate medical appointments. They often help with agitated residents who call or wander to the front desk. Savvy receptionists also serve as a sounding board for grieving families, screen callers, give clear and correct information and directions, and acknowledge callers and visitors courteously and promptly. Healthy organizations recognize the importance of the first impression and hire smart, likeable individuals who do not engage in personal calls, nail painting, and gossip with other employees.

Companies that have a standard of excellence train and reward their people. You can often discern whether or not it is a quality organization you are visiting by talking to the line staff (janitors, front desk, housekeepers, etc.). Service professions pay nominally, but some communities retain the same employees for years because they like to go to work and they are appreciated by management. They will loyally promote the community when you visit. The opposite is true for poorly run organizations.

SETTING THE APPOINTMENT

If you are calling an assisted living or nursing facility, ask to speak with the marketing director. Once you obtain the information that you need to proceed, you will be asked to set a tour date. The marketing director will likely want you to visit during business hours, but many of them also work weekends and you will want to return in the early evening or on a Saturday or Sunday to see how well things function on these off-times (there's always less staff and fewer managers then). Good communities run like clockwork seven days a week because competent supervisors attract quality people and thoroughly train shift leaders.

Ask the marketing director if the Executive Director or Administrator as well as the Director of Resident Care will be available during tour time. If not, reschedule or set a separate appointment. You need to be well acquainted with the people that are directly responsible for the care of your loved one, and you want to watch how they interact with one another. You need to observe the dynamic between these staff members because these are the ones who set the tone for the building.

If you are considering a small board and care home, you will get a very straightforward view of life in this residence as the lifestyle is far more informal and the owner is usually available. You need to meet day shift and overnight staff, so schedule these visits late in the afternoon as shifts change.

SNEAK A PEAK

Once you've set the tour, show up early. Walk the grounds. Observe back entrances. Are visitors trained to enter through front doors only? Do deliveries of goods to the facility seem to be monitored? Are people careful not to prop gates open? (Residents can be very manipulative and can convince an unsuspecting deliveryman that they need to exit). Do employees ensure that service providers close gates?

Approach a friendly-looking family member in the parking lot and ask if he would share his impressions of the facility with you. Most will be glad to.

Once you've entered the lobby, explain that you are early and would like to relax. Try to sit in an alcove nearby where you will be unnoticed and fade into the woodwork. Listen and observe. Do employees "hang around" the front desk and chitchat? Does the receptionist have projects to do? Is her work station tidy? How's her phone manner? If a resident trips an alarmed door, watch how the "rescue" process is conducted. Does the staff handle it calmly and efficiently?

Observe guests coming and going. Is the receptionist careful about having all visitors sign in and out? Do exiting family members seem pleased with their visits?

Are licenses and permits current and posted? How about the result for this year's state survey? Facilities in good standing will proudly display the results in a conspicuous spot near the front desk.******

******

****** All licensed facilities undergo an impromptu annual or semi-annual visit

In general, you should observe and experience a peaceful, orderly environment.

(survey) by the Department of Social Services liaison, whose job is to analyze records, procedures and the physical plant. This is a thorough inspection and minor flaws are noted for correction, while serious deficiencies result in possible citation, fines and the need for a follow-up visit. Ask to see the results of the survey. It's easy to discern if the problems are serious. You only want to consider facilities with perfect ratings or very minor, correctable deficiencies.

16

WHAT TO NOTICE ON TOUR

WHEN YOU TAKE YOUR tour, you'll want to note the **condition of the building** (inside and out), the **daily routines and activities** (including weekends), **safety and emergency procedures**, and the **relationship of staff to residents**, which reflects the overall philosophy of care exercised by the management. It is of utmost importance that you take the time to find out as much as you can about the leadership of the community.

Some readers may be surprised to find that little is mentioned about the physical presentation of the building. All you need to see is a clean building that offers safe and functional dining, activity and living areas. The tour of the grounds and facility is the icing on the cake. Your observations of the interpersonal relationships in the building and the interviews you will conduct with the staff are what will take up the vast majority of your appointment time.

You will notice that the largest percentage of the survey

questions pertain to the staff-resident relationship, followed by safety and building maintenance.

Be prepared to take a careful tour and make an appointment that should last at least one hour. You may bring this list along, and add any questions you deem appropriate. Do not apologize for your thoroughness – well-run facilities demonstrate the same degree of caution, and your job is to protect your loved one as best as you can.

CONDITION OF THE BUILDING

Are renovations occurring? How are these completed safely and with a minimum of disruption to the residents? Are cosmetic improvements taking precedence over areas that need practical attention? How about the back of the building? Are only the rooms in front being spiffed up?

Some residents have been lifelong smokers and continue to smoke. They are allowed to smoke in monitored outdoor areas. One community recently suffered a fire when a resident dropped a cigarette on her lap robe. Ask how the staff ensures safe smoking practices.

Are potentially dangerous games left unattended? Croquet stakes, golf holes, mallets may be left out and can cause trips and falls. Are there uneven or raised surfaces on paved walkways?

Some properties have large expanses of yard for residents to walk in. Are there corners or areas of the building that are not observed by cameras or staff? Could a resident fall and lie there for some time before being noticed?

Does the building smell fresh from front to back? Most residents battle incontinence and accidents are regular. The best facilities don't keep hampers in the residents' quarters – they merely collect soiled linens immediately and launder them. See what the policy is.

Ask to see the room where medications are stored. Some places show this on tour. This is where all records and medicines are stored and prepared for dispensing. Ask how the system works.

Could a medication be dropped or lost? Does the same person always hand out the medication? Are they strict about ensuring that the medication is given out within the time frame listed on the prescription? How do they handle it if a resident refuses to take the pill? Does the staff stick around to make sure that the pill is swallowed, or is the medication just handed out?

Where do visiting doctors, podiatrists, and psychiatrists examine residents? Is dignity and privacy observed? (I screened a facility once where the podiatrist was actually treating residents in the formal dining room!)

Are bathrooms clearly marked and easy for male and female residents to distinguish? Many don't have time to return to their room when they need to go. Who ensures that the resident is all right? How often does the janitorial staff check for wet floors after a resident visits the bathroom?

In older buildings ask staff about elevator use. Do residents operate it alone? How about those with unsteady gait? Who accompanies them? Stairs should be blocked. Many communities now are single-story, which eliminates that headache.

Handrails should be cleaned and disinfected regularly. Check on this.

DAILY ROUTINE

Do residents who wear glasses, hearing aids or dentures have these devices on every day? Lazy staff members do not take the time to ensure this. Is makeup on ladies light and natural or garishly applied? Have family received advice on appropriate clothing to bring for warm and cool seasons? Has the staff ignored the wool sweat suit that Mr. J. is wearing outdoors on a 90-degree day? Is Mrs. X. tottering around on high heels? How about Mrs. S. in that flimsy blouse, braless? (See Chapter 21)

Examine the posted activity calendar. Visit at varying times and make sure that the activities actually happen. Are the activities well-rounded? Do they seem childish or dignified? Residents should not be wearing ridiculous hats or singing babyish tunes. The instructor should be speaking clearly and slowly in order to be understood, but not in a patronizing manner. Residents with dementia are not children.

The activities should include walking and exercises, as well as interactive games and music. Music is particularly uplifting and residents who cannot participate should still be brought to the event. I have seen very confused residents get a spark of recognition or look of pleasure when they recognized a tune from the past. Many will remember a few bars or the melody of a patriotic song or classic hymn. Those who can sing will do so with some encouragement and enjoy it greatly.

Most communities take advantage of adult education courses, which cost only a few dollars a week to host. Do they offer pet therapy? This allows residents an outlet for cuddling and touching and the animals are well trained and gentle. Does the facility have a mascot? This allows high-functioning residents to participate in the feeding and care of the animal and to express physical affection. A resident garden is also helpful for those with extra energy.

Stay for a meal and observe. Do residents sit where they want or have assigned seating? What are the management's views on this? How do they determine the menus? Which types of snacks are available? What if Mom is too tired to come for a meal? What does the staff do when eating habits change?

Is everyone awakened and brought to meals and activities at the same time, or in shifts? Do the residents look clean? Does their hair appear washed and styled attractively? Are their outfits tidy and coordinated? It is to be expected that a resident will throw up or have an accident during the course of the day, and this should not surprise families. It is also reasonable to observe odd or inappropriate comments or behaviors, such as an outburst or even a resident walking out of his room naked. Staff cannot control these actions, and it happens in every facility. **What you want**

to see is how this is handled. Is staff quick to notice? Are they quiet and efficient? Do they make the resident wait unnecessarily? Do they rebuke or reassure? Barring these incidents, the tone of the facility should be calm and pleasant.

SAFETY AND EMERGENCY PROCEDURES

Does the facility perform head checks to ensure that all residents are accounted for? How frequently does this occur?

What's the policy in the event of fire or evacuation? Does each staff member have assigned duties and areas of the building to cover? What is the procedure?

Residents who wish to leave the community will often make a beeline for the outer gates or doors. Are these people redirected and noticed? Some individuals will linger in the hallways, confused. Are they walked back to an activity and comforted, or are they left to their own devices? Does the staff use gentle speaking tones or do they shout down the hallway at the person? Do caregivers escort the person by linking arms with them or do they pull them by the hand (like a wagon)?

Is the staff in uniform and wearing nametags? They need to be, as it helps reduce the chance of a resident perceiving the employee as a visitor or stranger and thus being unnecessarily frightened. Does kitchen staff wear hairnets? Are the hallways well lit and free from clutter or loud designs? Is there relaxing music played overhead or feverish rock tunes? Are floors clean with non-skid surfaces? Is carpeting frayed? Do the bathrooms have grab bars? Are cleaning carts (containing chemicals and solvents) or maintenance tools and equipment left in hallways unattended? Are long corridors punctuated with chairs and rest areas? Are forks or knives cleared away safely as soon as meals are finished?

Ask when mopping the floors is completed. Those yellow signs are not sufficient to keep a confused senior from walking into a newly mopped area. Mopping should be performed at night or in carefully blocked-off areas.

Are spills cleaned up immediately? Does the staff walk past the spill indifferently or do they handle it? If you sense an "It's not my job" attitude, take that seriously. This indicates management's willingness to allow employees to behave as though they are not part of a team and you can expect substandard care. These people negatively impact the morale of the staff and cast a pall over the community.

Is English spoken? Unless the community caters to a non-English speaking clientele, it is paramount that the staff speaks English in the presence of the residents. Good facilities enforce the policy, stressing to employees the spirit as well as the letter of the law. You need employees who can clearly understand what a resident is trying to communicate, especially since the senior may be in distress. It is also frightening to an already befuddled person to hear strange words spoken in a foreign tongue. Quality employees are anxious to please and will heed, though it may take some reinforcement on management's part as it is natural for people to lapse into their native language. Top-flight organizations educate and reward their employees for embracing "resident first" policies with a positive attitude.

Does staff pay attention when a resident is discharged to the hospital? Good facilities are ready for paramedics by having the resident's paperwork ready, and they ensure that the person does not go to the hospital dirty, unkempt, or cold. (Reception staff should be trained to make sure that busy EMT's (emergency medical technicians) do not take a resident out uncovered by a blanket (yes, it happens). EMT's sometimes are not experienced in recognizing dementia and may ask the resident questions ("Where does it hurt") which the person cannot understand. Ask if the facility uses a particular ambulance company and if the staff educates the EMT's.

STAFF/RESIDENT RELATIONSHIPS

First Things First

To gain insight into the type of staffing the facility offers, first *ask about the management company.*

Who is the management company and how long have they been in business? What is their philosophy of care? Do they have any involvement in the day-to-day operations or do they entrust everything to the executive director? You want a company that has a solid structure of accountability with a balance – enough to ensure that systems are in place without exercising too much presence and undermining the building's management. This is a tricky dance to execute. Corporations that exercise a "hands off' philosophy are foolish because they leave everything to the site manager. Good managers need support (to avoid burnout) and bad managers need training or dismissal. I have witnessed embezzlement, sexual scandals and large employee turnover occur as a result of corporate oversight.

Ask how many facilities they own. Some companies grow too fast and don't have the infrastructure to stretch that far. You don't want to settle your parent in a community that constantly changes hands. Ask if the building is owned or merely managed by the company, and if the latter, how long the management contract is for.

You can tell a lot about the company by the caliber of individual they choose as executive director. That individual should embody the philosophy of care the company believes in. Paper pushers or dictators either work for the same sort or are employed by people who don't have a clue about how to hire the right person for a job that requires tremendous "people skills."

Start at the Top

The director should be readily available, able to look you in the eye and not be someone who hides away in an office or pushes most of the work on subordinates. You need a director who is willing to take the time to confer with you about your parent's condition whenever you feel it warrants it. This administrator or executive director should be well connected in the medical community and have a good relationship with his licensing representative and the ombudsman, as well as several psychiatrists. Does the director have one or two reputable MD's who will make house calls or consult?

Does the director utilize a good gero-psych program in the area? Does she ensure that her director of resident care or director of nurses visits regularly and monitors daily any residents who are out of the facility at a hospital or other center? Is this person comfortable working with physicians who may not be proactive in helping your parent?

Ask about the director's background, licenses held and educational credentials. Find out if he has managed other local facilities and how many years he has worked in the industry. Does the person have a background in social services, nursing or related work or does he have a business background? Ideally you want someone who is savvy about the art of managing people and yet has service experience. The director needs to practice fiscal prudence to protect the company's financial interests but if his day is centered on "bottom line" matters then he is usually poor at leading a team. The director's administrative assistant should be the staff member who handles payroll, overtime issues, expenditures and monetary matters in order to free up the director to foster relations with staff, families and professionals. Meet the director's right-hand person – there is always such a person. Observe if they have complementary strengths.

How often does the director meet with staff? Many facilities hold a daily "flash meeting" for the management team to discuss relevant staffing and resident issues. Find out what is practiced in this facility. It is crucial that back-up management staff working nights and weekends have clear communication about the day-to-day concerns involving resident care and personnel issues.

Ask about census. The facility should be full with a waiting list, or fairly full (deaths always occur). If census is low, find out why. Sometimes there is a legitimate reason, like a company has assumed management of a badly run facility and has inherited low census. However, the occupancy should be building once the word gets out that the community is now stable. There is tremendous competition and facilities are in abundance in most metropolitan areas, so it is a little harder now to stay full, but the good places still manage to keep occupancy high.

What kind of relationship does the director have with the ombudsman? An ombudsman is a volunteer advocate that the public may notify to report suspected abuses or problems within the facility. The law requires that the phone number to the ombudsman be posted prominently in the facility. Contact the local ombudsman and ask if he would recommend a move to this particular establishment.

Who Cares?

By all means you will need to meet the director of resident care (in a nursing home, the director of nurses and in a board and care she is called the manager) before you make any decision about moving your loved one into a facility. Find out the type of training that this person has received. If she does not have a background in social work or nursing, she should at least have some certification in care for dementia, and a lot of practical experience. She should have a good reputation and relationship with several MDs whom she can call for advice or possibly house calls, as well as several good hospice and home care agencies. She should carefully monitor all resident health histories and be the liaison with the hospital or other center if the resident is sent out.

Ask how outbursts or violence is handled. Who handles disciplinary problems? Some residents can become extremely agitated due to the disease, reaction to medications, and various reasons. Is the staff calm and efficient in these emergencies?

Do they use behavior modification techniques of keeping the person stable before resorting to changing the meds?

This key staff member should be in frequent touch with families to inform them of emotional or physical changes of condition. She should have an efficiently organized medication room and a strong relationship with her caregivers, whom she trains on an ongoing basis. She should be vigilant about observing new challenges (chewing problems, depression) in her residents. She should be a confident advocate who would protect your loved one with the same commitment she would to her own relative. She should encourage your feedback as concerned family members.

How does she develop a care plan? How often is it revised? How about when a resident returns from a hospital visit?

Last But Certainly Not Least

While on tour you will want to watch closely the interaction between the line staff and the residents. When you are assembling your information from the director, you can ask about the staff. How are they hired? Have they had proper criminal clearance? I knew of a community that in one afternoon had to fire 10 employees who had supplied false social security documentation. If the director had proper systems in place this never would have occurred.

Does the company have a detailed manual of polices and procedures which are enforced and understood by employees? How frequently is the staff trained? Do subjects include emergency practices, sexual harassment, elder abuse and other relevant topics?

Are employees comfortable conversing with and handling confused residents who may become demanding? Are they trained to address the person respectfully and not in an overly familiar manner? Do they receive updates on new techniques, medications and ways of dealing with the dementia population? Do they understand that residents are not punished for bad behavior? Are they skillful at redirecting agitated residents and de-escalating tension? Are they resourceful in knowing how to convince a resident to take a shower or pill that he is resisting?

Does the employee buckle under pressure or does he seem good-natured and flexible? Does the company validate staff's hard work with awards and raises? Do employees seem to be treated as professionals with the respect and high expectations that accompany that distinction? Is there an incentive program? How are good employees acknowledged?

Ask about the ratio of staff to employees. Facilities that charge more will have more employees per residents (1 employee to 6 or 7 is considered good). For families whose loved one requires considerable supervision (frail, a fall risk, or a wanderer) – small board and care facilities are a good option as they offer more one-on-one contact. If finances permit, families can obtain a companion to come to the facility, as well.

If the facility is good-sized, ask if the employees are equipped with walkie-talkies. This is preferable, as staff frequently needs to summon one another in the event that there is an accident or other resident need or emergency.

How does management observe the overnight staff? How do they know if the graveyard shift is performing or sleeping on the job? Good companies conduct impromptu supervisory visits at all hours, install cameras, and assign tasks to overnight staff when they are not busy checking on residents. This helps ensure that staff members are not snoozing on a sofa when they need to be alert and safeguarding the building at night.

Older people generally require less sleep, and some residents will get up in the night and roam around. How does the staff handle this? Are residents hurriedly sent back to their rooms, or are they comforted and allowed to stay up for a while (which works better until the person relaxes). Does the staff patrol the building and check the grounds? Is the parking area well lit and any suspicious activity noted? Does the staff take advantage of "down time" by doing laundry or mopping floors, or is there a lot of TV watching going on at night? How about extra checks performed on residents newly arrived from a hospital stay? What special measures are taken?

By now you will certainly have formed a strong impression, one way or the other, as to whether this facility meets your needs or not. No facility is perfect, but you'll know if your loved one would be in good hands. Trust your instincts, and visit the facility one or two more times, if you need to. Bring some other family or a trusted friend. But take heart, for you are now expert at knowing how to glean much information, and if you need to keep looking your next tour will be much easier to undergo.

17

QUESTIONS FOR SKILLED NURSING ADMINISTRATORS

W HEN CONSIDERING ADMITTING YOUR loved one to an acute care/skilled nursing facility, you will want to have satisfactory answers to many questions. The best people from whom to obtain this information are the administrator of the facility and the director of nurses. Be sure to schedule an interview and allow time in which to discuss these points and any others with these professionals.

While the admissions representative or marketing director is the public's first point of contact and she may have a solid knowledge of the facility's operations, you need to meet with the management of the facility as they set the tone and enforce the philosophies and practices of patient care. Don't even consider a place that has an unavailable administrator.

Well-run facilities will be forthcoming in sharing information (hopefully before you need to ask). The following questions may be used in your meeting with the administrator.

BACKGROUND INFORMATION

- Who is your parent company? Do they own other facilities? Do they have a website I might access?
- What score did you receive on your most recent state survey? (You can see the results that are kept in a binder in the front lobby. Exemplary facilities proudly post "deficiency free" status).
- Do you have a medical director? What is his/her background and philosophy of care?
- Who is your ombudsman and what kind of relationship do you have with her? How about your licensing representative from the DSS? Would these professionals recommend a move to your facility?

STAFFING

- What is your ratio of staff to patients? Why?
- What do you do when you are short-handed for staff some days?
- Do you have a social worker on staff?
- Is there a house psychiatrist? Does he/she specialize in a particular discipline?
- Who manages the dementia program? What is his/her top priority?
- How often does staff receive training? Who conducts it? Are outside professionals involved?
- Is there a house doctor that you retain to attend patients, or is the patient's own physician called?
- What specific training does the staff have in handling dementia patients?
- Who is in charge in your absence? Are you on call?
- May I meet with the Director of Nursing?

PATIENT CARE

- What is your philosophy on patient care, particularly when dementia is a key factor?
- Is there a dietician on staff?
- Tell me how you accommodate special diets. Does your cook mind chopping up or pureeing food (some refuse to do this). Is your culinary staff knowledgeable about the dietary restrictions of those with dementia, especially in the latter stages of the disease? Who plans the meals?
- What is the policy regarding incontinence and toileting issues? Do you prefer to catherize? How often are patients changed and checked on?
- How does your staff handle angry or upset outbursts? What about depressed, withdrawn behavior?
- Is English spoken in the presence of patients? How strictly is this enforced? Are patients talked about as though they are not in the room, or spoken to in a childish or patronizing manner?
- How do you handle bed-bound patients and the accompanying problems such as bedsores?
- How frequently is the room cleaned?
- Will my loved one generally receive care from particular staff members, or do you rotate? Do you have staff that are skilled in serving those hard-to manage types of patients?
- Can you handle (if applicable) specific needs such as dialysis, Parkinson's disease or respiratory problems?
- What if my parent becomes terminally ill? Do you have a hospice program that you are affiliated with? What's the procedure?

DAILY ROUTINE

- Which type of regimen will the daily routine consist of?
- Are the programs appropriate by virtue of age and ability? Who plans them?
- How are they customized for dementia-related needs?
- What if my loved one is bedridden? Is there someone who would read/visit with her?
- Who manages the dementia program? What is his/her top priority?
- Are there activities in the evening or on the weekends? Who fills in for the program director in her absence?

FEES

- What are your fees? Does Medicare, insurance or other funding, cover these services?
- How about long-term policies or veterans' benefits?
- Please list all fees not covered, and likely extra charges.
- Do you have someone on staff that can assist in applying for little-known benefits for which we may be eligible for but are unfamiliar with?
- How frequently do you increase rates? (Expect them to quote an annual cost of living increase – ranges from 2-8%).
- Are there deposits required? What if my loved one is hospitalized or dies suddenly? Are any monies refunded?

EMERGENCY MEASURES

- What is your policy on the use of restraints? Some facilities restrain most of their patients as a time-saving measure. (This should not occur unless the person absolutely requires it for reasons of safety.)
- How does the staff handle a wanderer, particularly at night?

- At what point are psychoactive drugs used to manage agitated behavior?
- What is the policy about informing families of any change in condition, doctor visits, or related matters?
- If my loved one is hospitalized, who handles the follow-up? How frequently is she visited, and is the facility in daily contact with her doctor or social worker? (A must)
- Who contacts the family? Does a member of the staff visit my parent?
- What is your policy on life-sustaining measures?
- Which hospital do you use in an emergency? What's the procedure?
- What are your evacuation procedures? Are all staff members trained in them?

SAFETY ISSUES

- How is your dementia unit secured? Can a patient leave? What happens if he goes AWOL? Do patients hang around the doors or are they redirected?
- What is your visitor policy? Do you have specific hours?
- What if a roommate is violent or aggressive? Is my parent safe?
- How do you guard against theft or elder abuse?
- Who is responsible for evening and graveyard shifts? (Meet that person.)

FAMILY RELATIONS

- Do you offer families a forum in which they may discuss pertinent issues, receive updates, and interact with other families? Are there social functions held regularly at the facility?

- What recourse does the family have to express concerns or thoughts? Who are they directed to as a matter of policy?
- Do you have some family members of patients who would consent to speaking with me? (Live testimonials make the best referrals!)

In the natural course of conversation you may think of additional questions to pose to the staff. You should expect forthright, clear answers and an obliging attitude on the part of the representative. While the list may seem a bit daunting, it is important to remember that winning organizations will respect your cautious and thorough approach.

18

AVOIDING
INAPPROPRIATE
PLACEMENT

BEWARE WHEN FACTS SAY one thing and emotions (or people) say another.

Reputable facilities want – in fact, insist upon – appropriate placement. They know that for the good of the client and in fairness to the family and the staff an honest assessment and sometimes a declined admittance is the ethical thing to do. Nothing is worse than the trauma of uprooting and moving a loved one into a facility that is ill-equipped to handle the person.

Early in my career, I watched as many facilities became licensed to offer additional services, coined "assisted living." These services generally included bathing, dressing, and medication management. Admission criteria included completion of a physician's report (which provided a current overview of the client's health). Licensing regulations prohibited facilities from admitting residents with a ***primary diagnosis*** of dementia. Only facilities with a dementia waiver could admit residents with such a diagnosis.

Some census-challenged communities that do not serve a dementia population have attempted to convince families that they can care for a senior who is physically okay but afflicted with dementia. Families are urged to ask the doctor to change the primary diagnosis to a secondary one, so that the resident may move in to the community. This is a paperwork game and unfortunately occurs in some struggling communities that need the revenue and who may feel pressure to play with the diagnosis in order to admit your parent legally into the facility. Beware of this, and keep in mind that people who cut corners in important issues like this likely have questionable standards in other ethical considerations, too. Doctors do not usually affix a dementia diagnosis to someone with mild, age-related forgetfulness. It is likely that the primary diagnosis is correct.

Obviously, the practice of "diagnosis switching" is wrong for many reasons. Not only is the facility downplaying the need for your loved one to get appropriate care, but they are not factoring the added strain that a poor placement will put on the family, the staff, and most of all, the resident. The facility may assert that your parent is in the early stages of dementia, that the staff can handle his needs, and you may be convinced that a move to a dementia facility would be premature.

HOW TO DETERMINE IF DEMENTIA CARE IS NEEDED

Families faced with the choices of placement of their loved one in an independent assisted living community as opposed to a specialized dementia/assisted living program naturally will wish that their parent could function in the former setting. No one wants his relative to live with others who are confused, and some family members mistakenly believe that if their loved one is exposed to "with-it" seniors he might respond well. Families struggling with denial of the disease may be tempted to concede to pressure to give an independent community a try, hoping that Mom will "get better." This is understandable, and I feel very sympathetic to this response, but families who deny a dementia diagnosis are asking for trouble. Moving a senior into a community in which she cannot function adequately is unfair to the individual, the other residents, and the staff. This usually results in one or more scenarios, such as:

- **Short tenancy**, often fraught with problems. The natural period of acclimation and adjustment are replaced with a series of frustrating mishaps and unmet expectations.

- **Possible eventual eviction** due to inability of client to function independently in accordance with community expectations. For instance, resident will forget meals, hoard food, behave inappropriately towards others (sexual advances, verbal outbursts, bizarre mode of dress); cannot participate in daily routines.

- **Withdrawal from population** as a result of inability to communicate or interact with others; isolation. Delays in addressing this behavior increase the likelihood for the development of depression, along with the likelihood of an accident, injury or related crisis.

- **Indifferent or unkind treatment by residents** While some seniors will be sympathetic to the confused individual, many will feel uncomfortable and will steer clear of the person. They will likely gossip to others and complain to management. Confused residents may be ostracized in the dining room, especially if they are unable to keep up with conversations and have indelicate table manners. Residents also have little patience watching staff help feed or wipe the mouths of those unable to care for themselves.

- **Poor care** Employees (even very good caregivers) need special training to handle those with dementia (since physical and behavioral changes are common). Staff need to allot their time differently in caring for this population, and must possess specific interactive and problem-solving skills in addition to those involving medication, bathing and dressing assistance.

- **_Greater exposure to financial and other abuses_** While assisted living communities do screen visitors, they are not secured facilities and residents have their own schedules, usually have a private telephone, and can entertain guests with few restrictions. Confused seniors can walk out the door, call a cab, or be preyed upon by an unscrupulous telemarketer or new "friend" fairly easily.

WHAT YOU CAN DO

If you doubt the dementia diagnosis, have your parent re-examined. Review the testing procedure with the physician. Have additional testing performed by a geriatric psychiatrist. Get a professional opinion as to whether your parent needs a specialized program or not. If you again receive a primary diagnosis of dementia, do not move your parent into any facility lacking proper qualifications for dementia care.

THE IMPORTANCE OF DETAILED ASSESSMENTS

As mentioned earlier, the question may be raised about moving your parent to a dementia facility prematurely. Remember that a good program will thoroughly assess your loved one to make sure that he would be well served. Some dementia programs cater to the newly diagnosed types while others serve mid-to-late stage clients. The right program will match your loved one with roommates, table mates and other companions who are compatible.

CHANGED EXPECTATIONS

Don't forget that if your loved one truly suffers from dementia, she will not be looking critically at the things that matter to the rest of us. Her expectations will not be the same, and she will not care about details like room size, décor and appointments, and availability of salad bars at mealtimes. In many ways, the person has assumed childlike, egocentric characteristics in that her needs are simple and of utmost importance. If she is fed, comfortable and cared for, she will be okay. Meaningful friendships, possessions, and values, which others hold, have ceased to be a consideration in the world of a confused person.

ADDITIONAL THINGS YOU CAN DO

1) **Visit** the non-dementia facility during meals and activity times. Ask yourself if your parent could function and fit in well. Imagine that your parent has no assistance. Would he have the ability to summon help in the middle of the night? Would he be able to evacuate in an emergency – on his own?

2) **Ask** to meet the president of the Resident Association. This individual is usually quite representative of the resident population as a whole, and he will often accurately reflect the tone of the facility. While some facilities serve a more sedentary group of seniors and others attract the active set, both factions pride themselves on not being "old people." Quiz this individual and ask yourself if your parent could hold his own at a resident meeting or outing.

3) **Arrange** for the Director of Resident Care to conduct an informal "interview" (assessment) of your parent. Do not answer any questions and don't let the DRC lead her into responding. If your parent is generally unaware of her whereabouts and the responsibilities of living in a community, then you have your answer.

For those reluctant family members who still need convincing, obtain a copy of the move-in agreement. If your parent can't read, understand, explain or sign it, than you know this would be an inappropriate placement. Make the correct arrangements and comfort yourself with the knowledge that the things that you wish were more attractive about specialized care mean nothing to your loved one.

Chapter 19 will be of assistance to those who are satisfied with the information received, but who need that final "push" to make a move a reality.

19

ENLISTING THE AID OF
THE DOCTOR

MARY R. (A PHYSICIAN, herself, by the way) was a woman
I consulted with. She attempted to convince a reluctant
parent to move his spouse into a care facility when it was clearly
needed. Mary was at a disadvantage because her parents lived in
another state. Mom had Alzheimer's. Mary and her siblings were
continually frustrated that Dad would drag his feet about getting
help. Mom had had a few close calls, and a neighbor had notified
Adult Protective Services. Mom went to a nursing home for a few
days, and Dad began to realize that perhaps he couldn't adequately
care for her anymore. His fright at her hospitalization made him
more vulnerable to direction. The ball was dropped, though,
because the family did not seize their golden opportunity. Mom
was discharged after a two-day hospital stay and Dad promptly
returned her home.

Mary realized too late that she missed her chance. **She didn't
enlist the aid of the doctor.**

THOUGHTS ON THE ROLE OF THE PHYSICIAN

A key supporting player who should be actively involved in bringing about a change in care is the family physician. Most are conscientious and usually quite willing to oblige, as they are committed to their patient's best interests. They feel sympathetic to the well spouse's struggle and are aware of the declining health of their patient. They know that a facility or care program will be able to provide needed support, as they have other patients who have benefited from similar arrangements.

Physicians have tremendous demands on their time, but it only takes a few moments for them to exercise their greatest asset – a sense of authority. Keep in mind that many people over the age of 70 have a lifetime of viewing medical doctors with a sense of deference and respect. Doctors may be advising essentially the same actions that you are recommending, but they can expect full credibility for these reasons:

- Physicians fulfilled multiple roles before the advent of the many specialties existing today. The medical model was largely represented by the family practitioner who doubled as therapist and counselor before those disciplines were commonplace. An air of mystique and exclusivity surrounded the white-collar medical profession. Doctors (along with judges and pastors) were voices of authority largely for the rest of society, and were treated as such. These attitudes passed from generation to generation and many seniors today still show tremendous deference to the opinions of their physicians.
- Women (who made up the biggest percentage of patients) traditionally were especially encouraged to defer to authority figures. A doctor's word was law. Questioning a diagnosis was impolite.
- Few people in past decades had the level of education of their physician, and felt unqualified to debate a diagnosis or etiology of a disease, let alone participate in care-related decisions.

WHAT IF MY PARENT AVOIDS DOCTORS?

Some family members I have worked with confided that their loved one had a deep distrust for doctors and thus avoided them. In these cases, it is best to arrange for a home health nurse to come to the house for an evaluation. If the "well spouse" is part of the problem, you will probably need to involve Adult Protective Services if the spouse or senior refuses necessary medical care. At that point you can enlist the aid of a family law attorney or other professional who can help you.

Side note – In the case of adult children like Mary, it is highly advisable that an outside physician be engaged to handle all medical directives and related matters and operate as the senior's primary physician. Mary's relationship to her parents was perceived on both sides as that of a daughter who was also a physician. Her credibility with her father and the necessary detachment and authority she needed were compromised simply because of her status as a family member. This is a natural by-product of the family dynamic and I have witnessed this in many instances. Unfortunately, precious time was lost that might not have been if only the physician son or daughter didn't try to serve as the family doctor.

SETTING THE STAGE

Most family members, though, will consent to a visit to the doctor, so set the stage for a successful appointment which can yield you additional support and give your relative the push needed to move into the next phase of care. If the doctor has already tried to convince the caregiver or senior to take steps, this visit will serve to reinforce what has already been said. The doctor's time restraints, though, don't allow him much room for follow-up. Therefore, nothing has happened. The difference, though, is that **this** visit will produce results, because you, the advocate, will guide the process.

PRESCRIPTION FOR SUCCESS

Your first step is to contact the office manager and arrange for an immediate evaluation. Here's what you do:

1) Call early in the morning and ask for the office manager. Give her your parent's name and explain the seriousness of your parent's situation, and your fears. (If there is a well spouse in the picture, discuss his/her shame and reluctance in seeking help.) If the senior lives by himself, convey to the office manager the degree of dementia and the danger the person faces at home.

2) Explain that you need the manager to assist you in enlisting the doctor's cooperation. Usually you will find that the office staff is already aware of the problem (if parent has been receiving regular care). Sometimes the office manager will inform families that the doctor has already expressed concern or even recommended precautionary measures.

3) Ask the office to contact the patient (if she is still high-functioning enough to comprehend) or spouse to say that records show it is time for a check-up. If one was completed recently, the office can substitute an excuse (more tests needed, etc.). In more desperate situations, I have recommended that the manager state that the doctor has requested that the patient come in as he feels the need to review some information at this point in time. Explain to the office manager how you would like the appointment to unfold, by outlining this and the following steps.

4) The office can set it up to give a very brief, cursory exam. The goal is for doctor to explain that the patient is exhibiting alarming deterioration (they are very good at this and will usually find an existing condition to extrapolate from – i.e. diabetes, poor gait, etc.)

5) Once a brief exam has been conducted, the doctor can share with the family that he has concluded from his observations that the senior must immediately receive additional help to combat this rapid decline. The doctor can now introduce the literature and resource information (that you supplied in advance of the appointment) as he makes his recommendations.

6) The doctor can next inform the families that he would like placement in a respite program immediately following TB clearance and completion of an assessment. He can explain that he knows of a top-notch facility and that a bed is available. (He knows this because you have already confirmed this with the director of the facility.) The doctor can explain that he is recommending a 60-day respite stay at a retirement community so that the senior can be monitored carefully and concentrate on building his strength. Even if the senior has no outstanding condition save for the dementia, the doctor can still emphasize that the respite program can offer lots of rest, activity and good meals, along with specialized activities that can help the person remain connected to others.

(Whether or not you intend to keep your loved one at home and retain home health care, I strongly recommend that you attempt a respite stay in order to drive home the seriousness of the situation, give the caregiver a break, help stabilize the senior's health, and usher in the transitional stage with the support of others.)

7) The next step is for the nurse or office manager to arrange for a facility representative to perform an assessment that day. This will not be a problem because you will have already made these arrangements and the director of resident care will be awaiting the call. Most facilities will be happy to perform the assessment at a residence, doctor's office or hospital setting.

If the facility is located some distance away, ask the liaison if she can arrange for a representative from a local sister facility to perform an assessment (most facilities are part of a chain and can usually accommodate this request). If there are no affiliates in your area, the assessment will need to be performed on the day of admission.

Before you panic and wonder what happens if she doesn't pass the assessment, be aware that while there are some cases of those who experience sudden health declines, this scenario will likely not occur. The Director of Resident Care can review all pertinent health information to make sure that the admission is appropriate.

Unless the senior significantly fails during the trip to the facility, there should be no surprises. You will confirm this by already understanding what the requirements for admission are and reviewing these with the medical staff.

Besides, you will have already checked out and lined up an available bed in a quality nursing facility (just in case).

8) Now it is time for the doctor to inform the caregiver that he will monitor the success of the respite visit by having his nurse schedule a follow-up appointment when the stay is over. Many doctors make house calls and a growing number of facilities have on-site medical clinics for visiting physicians to utilize, or you can simply arrange for a follow-up appointment at the MD's office. If your loved one is moving out of the area, you can work with the DRC to switch your parent to a physician that has a relationship with the facility. Let the DRC know to which health plan the senior belongs to and ask for recommendations. Make sure that the new physician feels comfortable treating seniors with dementia and that the facility can transport your parent to regular office visits.

9) The doctor will next supply the well spouse with information (that you again have provided) to help *her* learn about support groups, weekend guest programs at independent retirement communities, helpline and resource information, as well as a color brochure of the facility providing the respite stay and details describing its dementia program.

Keep in mind that the word "moving" is not being discussed at this point. Unless the senior is very passive and the well spouse is completely agreeable, it is better to present these suggestions as part of a temporary intervention brought on by medical necessity. This allows the well spouse to come to terms with the need for permanent change while learning to let go of feelings of guilt. There are no strings attached and this approach allows the doctor to be the "heavy." It works beautifully when handled properly and I have counseled hundreds of families to employ this method – with successful results. In most cases the transition was uneventful and the caregiver relieved.

IS THIS DUPLICITOUS?

Some may feel that this approach is duplicitous, unfair or disrespectful to the senior or the caregiver. However, if the situation is at crisis point and you believe that some intervention is necessary because the senior's safety is at stake, you must re-evaluate. If the doctor's appointment is handled diplomatically, order can be re-established in a rapidly worsening situation. Dozens of families I have worked with can back up this assertion.

Remember that the doctor is not forcing this move – just merely urging it. The well spouse can certainly opt to keep the person home, provided she exercises a viable plan of care (see chapter on home care). In my experience, this exhausted, depressed caregiver nearly always consents to the trial respite stay. The doctor's insistence is often the push that the spouse needs. She has merely wanted permission.

Once the well spouse consents, it is of the utmost importance to move quickly, so a form of "buyer's remorse" doesn't set in. This does not mean that the spouse is not given a thorough and realistic overview of the program, nor does it mean that her feelings are to be overlooked. It means that this is a very emotional time and the hand-off must be effortless or the game will be over before it has been played.

RE-ESTABLISHING ROLES QUICKLY

After the successful visit to the doctor, arrange to have the well spouse phoned and personally invited by the executive director to meet at the facility. Both the director and the resident care director will need to guide this meeting, anticipate the nervousness and possible guilt and be prepared to re-focus the person's energies on *being an active part of the care plan.*

It is imperative that the program is presented as a *supportive and supplemental service* in conjunction with the doctor's care plan. The well spouse needs to be informed that her role is key to the success of the program, as she knows the patient better than anyone else. In addition to completing the admission and health information, she should be polled on a variety of subjects and asked questions about her husband's quirks, habits, and preferences, as well as any suggestions she may have for care. Her inclusion in this vital discussion will determine her level of cooperation for the remainder of her spouse's tenancy. The spouse should be made to feel that the facility is an ally who respects her influence and will appreciate any input she can give. If she views the staff in this light, she will transition smoothly and consent to admission.

20

SETTLING IN

AS YOU PREPARE TO move into the facility, you will need to bring the appropriate items and make sure that the room is ready for occupancy.

- Nowadays, large facilities and nearly all board and care homes supply a furnished room. (If they do not, you will need to bring a single bed and a few pieces of furniture). Here are a few pointers to help you as you get ready to move your loved one's belongings:
- Beds in facilities may only have a half-rail. A doctor's order will allow you to obtain this protective device from a medical supply store. If your loved one is in danger of tumbling out of bed, ensure that this item is ordered and that one side of the bed is placed securely against a wall (if possible). Check to see if licensing regulations in your state allow the box spring to be removed and the mattress placed on a flatter surface, closer to the floor.
- Make sure that the care plan reflects the need for night staff to check periodically (especially in those first few weeks) to see that your parent is tucked in securely. Night lights are

helpful but should be discreetly placed so that the tenant does not fixate on or is bothered by the glare.

- Check to see whether you supply the toiletries or if the facility includes them. Most of the time, the toilet paper, linens and towels are provided and laundered by the facility (especially in nursing homes). Make sure that shampoos, lotions, and other sundries are stored securely. There should be designated locked boxes or cabinets in the rooms for this purpose. (You don't want Dad making a cocktail with available cologne).

- You will not need to worry about bringing many belongings because most residents share modest-sized rooms. Resist the urge to bring tired knick-knacks – they will hold little meaning for the confused individual and usually disappear after a period of time. Some communities affix a "shadow box" (usually at the front door of the room), which contains photos and some mementoes. With this exception, it is wise to leave sentimental treasures with the family. Bring a few photographs, and leave the rest at home. (Many communities now arrange to post in the shadow box or on the door a mini-biography and affix it with a flattering photograph of your loved one. While this will mean little to your parent, it is a respectful gesture which helps reinforce to staff and visitors that the resident has his own history.)

- Do NOT bring the crown jewels. Residents will hide, flush, or give them away more often than not. Again, these possessions usually mean little to the confused person. If you must, replace Mother's wedding diamond with a cubic fake and keep the real thing at home. Don't risk theft or loss of a valued heirloom.

- Label everything. Because many residents are incontinent, items are frequently laundered and they can get mixed up and returned to the wrong person.

- Televisions are usually allowed, but unless the senior is very high functioning and can follow this activity, the set will sit untouched. Most facilities provide viewing areas in the common area lounges, and remember that the goal of good programs is to keep the resident OUT of his room most of the day. In addition, hearing problems coupled with memory loss can present conflicts if there is a roommate with whom to contend. Residents also get frustrated trying to work the television, are confused by the dials, and may attempt to "fix" the TV (often disabling it or harming themselves in the process). This advice also applies to the use of radios, microwaves or other electronic goods.
- Make sure that trash and laundry is picked up daily. To avoid contamination and odor, soiled bedding, garments and underclothes should be detected and collected by housekeeping, maintenance and caregivers on a daily basis, as well.

Side Note – Efficient, caring administrators not only cross-train their staff, but also direct all employees in learning how to spot potential problems before they arise. A maintenance man repairing a resident's broken air conditioner should notice smells from a dirty hamper and report them. The same thing goes for a laundress or kitchen helper who may be in the hallway and sees a resident outburst or accident. Staff should know how to defuse the situation and promptly summon management.

SAFETY AND CONVENIENCE FEATURES

Check to see if the tub or shower is properly equipped with grab bars and non-skid surfaces. If residents do not have a private bath, check to see how showering and toileting are completed.

(Your care plan should review mom's pre-admission routines and note special needs or longstanding habits. Examples of this would include "usually resists showers at night," "hates getting up early" or "prefers female attendants.") You will want caregivers to try to simulate meal and showers as reasonably close to the current routine as possible. Does Mom have incontinence? Make sure the schedule factors in regular toileting checks, the staff notifies you of changes and that protective garments are in stock at all times. Does the community re-order them and bill you for the cost, or are you responsible to notice if the supply is running low? Has a low toilet been modified with a commode? Would your parent feel self-conscious being bathed or dressed by a male caregiver? Make sure this is taken into consideration.

LOCATION, LOCATION, LOCATION

What does the room look out on? If it faces the outside of the property, check to see if the windows are tinted or one-way, or if the view is obstructed by drapes or blinds. Can anyone look into the room? Are the drapes drawn nightly? If this is a ground-floor room, check to see if there is an access door to the grounds (older buildings or converted apartments have these). Doors should be permanently locked to prevent someone from entering from the outside, as well as your loved one exiting. If your parent is a wanderer, request or get on the wait list for a room that does not face the street as this may fuel the desire for escape. All second-story rooms should have securely fastened windows. Ask for a room with a garden view if your parent tends to be excitable or frightened of strangers. Families may reason that the senior would enjoy watching deliverymen, visitors and activity, but overlook the fact that a confused individual could easily be aggravated about seeing unknown persons coming to "my house."

STAFF AWARENESS

- Ask the activity director how residents are summoned for classes and activities. The employees need to bring EVERYONE who is not ill or sleeping out of their rooms each day. It is paramount that residents be connected with events, people, and the energy of the community – regardless of their ability to contribute or function.
- Find out from the staff how they keep curious residents from exploring other's rooms.
- Although rooms are equipped with call systems for emergencies, most residents do not have the ability to summon assistance. Ask how the facilities handle this problem.
- Regular "Family Night" and other interactive activities are very helpful in keeping healthy dialogue open between the administration and the families. While luaus, themed events and parties are enjoyable, it is essential that a facility also offer informational evenings with updates on company news, legislation that may impact this population, and general "housekeeping" topics involving the day-to-day operation of the facility. Be sure to attend these meetings, or, if the facility does not offer one recommend that such a forum be held quarterly.

Keep in mind that because there are no resident councils in skilled nursing facilities, and that a good portion of the population may not have an active family advocate, it is doubly important to be vigilant in ensuring excellent care for your loved one. Your attentiveness will not only benefit your relative, but others as well.

21

CLOTHING GUIDELINES

Packing clothing for a move is easy, as there will be neither room nor necessity for many outfits. (You can still use these tips if your parent is remaining at home, as his needs have shifted and you may want to make a fresh start with a functional, up-to date wardrobe).

To ensure that your parent has what he needs, it is best to follow these simple guidelines:

HOW MUCH TO BRING

Pack 15 changes of clothing. Remember that frequent washings will create the need for regular replacement of undergarments and outfits. Rule of thumb: check the durability of the garment every six months – or when you rotate your warm weather outfits out for winter clothing.

BEST BETS

Choose outfits that can withstand regular laundering (cotton blends, polyester, etc.) Be aware that scratchy fabrics can be a source of irritation to delicate skin.

Avoid high-maintenance ensembles unless you plan to hand-wash or dry-clean the clothing on a regular basis. Bear in mind that shaky hands and inattention to detail create spills and spots on outfits.

Select flattering shades and try to choose solid colors for greater mix-and-match possibilities. This will help the staff greatly.

Don't overwhelm a petite lady with loud prints and large designs. Choose modest, delicate patterns.

Don't bring tired old clothing. Dad is not going to have any sentimental attachment to the baggy pair of pants or faded shirt he has worn a million times. Maintain his dignity with garments that are comfortable and appropriate.

Respect your parents' clothing preferences. If mom always wore dresses, pack these. If dad was conservative in his tastes, select comfortable outfits that are simple and functional but resemble his classic style.

Label everything. Due to the high volume of laundering that is done throughout the day, it is easy for clothing to get mixed up.

UNDERWEAR

Pack several new, labeled bags of soft, thick socks.

Some women may resist wearing brassieres. Purchase the sport-type, which are very hard to remove. Replace undergarments regularly and make sure that bras are supportive, particularly those for well-endowed women. Invest in quality bras that are not thin and lacy.

SPECIAL NEEDS

Choose pants with no pockets if your loved one has gait problems. You do not want the person shoving his hands into the pockets and risk losing his balance when walking. These pants are especially useful if your loved one has a tendency to hoard food or "borrow" items in the facility.

Order a catalog or go online for clothing that is especially created for this frail population. You will find an assortment of under and outerwear, in addition to shoes and useful accessories, such as attractive cummerbund-style bibs that can be worn at mealtime.

Residents that tend to want to remove clothing throughout the day do well if they wear suspenders and garments secured by a belt. If the senior does not have this tendency, he may wear pull-up, elastic-waist trousers. These are comfortable and require little time to remove or put on (again, a help to the caregiver).

Be realistic about accidents. Loss of control is a common by-product of dementia, but it doesn't have to be a problem. If you suspect incontinence, provide some lightweight pad or briefs. Make sure the bed has protective plastic padding.

FOOTWEAR

See that shoes have rubber soles and if the resident is a woman, ditch the high heels. No sight is more chilling than to see a senior wobbling onto a jerky elevator or walking on a flagstone garden path in pointy pumps. If the resident tends to remove shoes, choose comfortable shoes that need tying or fastening. Otherwise, provide slip-on or Velcro-strap shoes to aid a busy caregiver as she dresses your parent. Bring a simple pair of tennis shoes or loafers for a man. If the woman is steady on her feet, include very low, thick-heeled shoes or espadrilles to go with a nice dress.

Often in the evenings residents like to wander about in slippers. You can purchase slippers that are durable and not lightweight. Keep in mind that they should be thick enough to withstand stepping on a sharp or pointed object.

Your loved one may rebel against wearing glasses, hearing aids and dentures. Make sure that they fit properly and comfortably. Confirm that the staff logs these items as inventory and remind them to urge your parent to wear them every day.

TOILETRIES

Don't forget Dad's shaving kit and nose hair trimmers. Make sure that the beautician or caregivers take care of this on a regular scheduled basis, or set some time aside on your visits to make sure this important grooming ritual happens. Check hair in the ears as well.

If you provide special soaps or shampoos, make sure that they are not harsh to the skin. Most residents do not shower daily because of the frequency of skin breakdowns. Thus, it is important that the staff is instructed to apply powder, deodorant and other fresh-smelling beauty aids to the resident daily.

Make sure that you keep toothpaste and mouthwash stocked, and double-check to ensure that the staff is using it regularly. Has the mouthwash sat untouched for months? Pay attention.

Most ladies wore and still like makeup. Include some inexpensive cosmetics that are hypoallergenic and soft in color. Throw out any red lipsticks and blue eye shadow and make sure that the caregiver who helps mom apply makeup does not overdo it. Your mother's dignity must be maintained at all times and nothing is more pathetic than to see an elderly resident with clownish makeup.

OTHER GROOMING IDEAS

Hair does not require daily washing, but should be neatly combed and in place. Pack a soft, natural bristle brush (to discourage pulling hair), and a wide-toothed comb. If mom's hair is long, include some simple, dignified clips or barrettes.

Most facilities have a beauty shop. Consult the beautician about flattering, easy wash-and-wear hairstyles. Short hair on women is recommended unless the resident has the ability and interest in caring for her hair (which seldom occurs). Don't, though, let the beautician whack off mom's hair into a boyish cut just to simplify things. Go for a short cut, but include for the staff some hair spray or gel for a quick morning styling. If mom can endure the process and her scalp won't be irritated, get a permanent and buy a few months of easy hair care. Many women receive pleasure from sitting under a hair dryer – perhaps this triggers a dim happy memory of past experiences.

If you can afford it and your parent can sit through it, arrange for a manicure and pedicure on a regular basis. Most facilities have a visiting podiatrist who makes house calls about once a month. If your parent is fidgety, try to do a quick trim job on one of your visits. Residents can scratch themselves if nails go untended.

MISCELLANY

Keep the amount of jewelry to a minimum, and do not pack authentic gems. Costume jewels will suffice for a lady who enjoys wearing them, and are inexpensive to replace if the items are lost, thrown out or given away (a common practice). Most residents with dementia pay little attention to jewelry, and have ceased to remember the significance of a wedding ring or other heirloom. If, however, your loved one is in the early stages of dementia and might still have an attachment to a special piece, keep the original gem safely at home and substitute a good fake.

Many seniors get cold easily due to circulatory problems and less output of energy. Heavy sweaters are inappropriate for the hot months, but make sure that you provide a nice lightweight sweater or windbreaker for afternoons in the garden.

Make certain that warm outfits are put away in summer months, and vice-versa. I would be infuriated if I saw my loved one meandering along on a hot day in a heavy Pendleton shirt. Ask the staff to make sure that inappropriate outfits are stored out of sight until the right time.

Help the caregiver by grouping outfits in the closet, and color-code accordingly. A hurried caregiver will appreciate your thoughtfulness in helping her dress your loved one on a rushed morning.

Now, maybe more than ever, is it important for your loved one to face the world with as much dignity as possible.

22

SPIRITUAL CARE

PEOPLE WHO LET GO of life, whether suddenly or slowly – do so because their world lacks hope. Hope – that great motivator, must be seen as real, attainable, and accessible to everyone, regardless of his situation, ability or qualities. Without hope, the world is colorless and life stretches on monotonously. Our incentive for living slips away.

The essence of our human makeup consists of three intertwined elements – our body, soul and spirit. To care for our physical selves, to shape and nurture the development of the mind, will and emotions (soul) but to overlook the needs of the spirit is to ignore a vital component of who we are. We shortchange ourselves of the healing benefits that come from having our spirits fed and ministered to. Consequently, it becomes difficult to maintain hopeful expectations for our lives.

DON'T OVERLOOK YOUR SPIRITUAL NEEDS

Our spirit, that life force that transcends our physiological limitations, is often downplayed or outright ignored by our increasingly cynical culture. Today's "advanced thinking" places great emphasis on the tangible – the obvious. After all, it **is** easier to identify physical or even emotional problems than to address spiritual needs. There is an abundance of "how-to" books, programs, and television shows that offer advice on nearly every aspect of the mental, physical and emotional sides of the human state. Uppermost in our mind then, is the need to take care of these aspects of our being. However, people forget that spiritual imbalance negatively impacts our functioning in these other areas of our lives. Don't underestimate your need for spiritual strengthening and encouragement in this time of trial.

A holistic approach to the problem can aid families who are facing the dilemma of dementia. As they put a plan of action in place in order to regain equilibrium in their lives and effective care for their loved one, caregivers will find greater satisfaction if they allot time daily to the pursuit of spiritual peace. This means taking regular periods in each day to devote to prayer, introspection and quiet time with God. Delve into teachings that can help you with your struggles and gain insight into your nature. Attend worship services whenever possible, even if you are tired or discouraged.

Years ago my music teacher discussed a fascinating study that compared those who sang hymns and songs of praise on a regular basis to those who did not. The former group consistently demonstrated a greater capacity for quicker healing and/or greater immunity from illness. In addition, the psychological benefits from corporate worship in a variety of cultures have also been well documented over the decades. In his writings on "Mental Health Ministry of the Local Church" (Abdington Press), Howard J. Clinebell Jr. wrote "studies in the psychology of music show that group singing is an effective way of creating group solidarity." Connection with others is key to the well-being of any person, and particularly those laboring under heavy burdens.

SPIRITUALITY AND DEMENTIA

People may assume that when an individual's cognitive functioning is severely compromised that his spirituality wanes or vanishes as well. Consequently, little value is often attached to addressing the person's spiritual needs on a continual basis. Just as it is important to make sure the senior is receiving regular meals, it is equally crucial to not withdraw his spiritual food.

CAN PEOPLE WITH DEMENTIA BE REACHED SPIRITUALLY?

People argue this question, and some assert that it is hard enough to measure reasoning power in one with dementia, let alone his receptivity to matters of the spirit (therefore, they assume, a waste of effort). While this perspective is understandable, my experience and that of countless pastors, counselors, and family members that I have interacted with over the years would disagree. One might contend that the examples provided are anecdotal and that we really have limited scientific means by which to measure spiritual response (although more attention and research is being directed towards the relationship between spirituality and dementia).

My response to this skepticism is this – that spirituality, which deals with the infinite and the intangible by definition cannot be measured with a scientific yardstick, and secondly, why deprive an individual the opportunity to participate in a reverent, worshipful service conducted by caring individuals? At worst, the senior would observe a peaceful assembly and be untouched; at best he would be stimulated on some level and respond in kind.

I believe your goal should be to provide an isolated, confused and perhaps frightened individual an opportunity to experience corporate worship and receive the benefits that flow from that. ***Our spirit cannot be confined***, which I believe is the key element of hope for all that have been bound by this terrible disease. The person with dementia, for once, is not inferior to any other in attendance at a worship service, as this is the one realm in which we are all equals. He or she also is not limited to a finite degree of comfort typically measured, documented and controlled.

AMAZING GRACE

Many facilities include worship services in their weekly activity regimen, which are usually conducted by visiting rabbis, ministers and lay clergy. Some communities offer communion services and some have volunteers who periodically gather to pray with residents, sing hymns and visit. If your parent lives in a facility that does not have much of a spiritual program, discuss with the director how one might be developed. If your parent still resides at home, contact your local house of worship to see if pastoral visits can be arranged, or inquire if the church offers specialized services as described in the following paragraph.

The Alzheimer's Association created an Interfaith Outreach Program that serves to connect families of those with Alzheimer's with specialized religious programs in the community. The advantage of this program is that arrangements are made by participating houses of worship for the senior to attend a service in the church or synagogue. The benefits of this, explains Jean Moonilal, Care Consultant of the Orange County Chapter of the Alzheimer's Association, are that "seniors often find these visits evoke early memories – the stained glass windows, the baptismal font, incense, the Torah. Certain sights and smells and a certain sense of reverence and sanctity cannot be duplicated. We have seen people who haven't spoken in years chanting along with the cantor or singing hymns, sometimes to the amazement of their children who came along with them." Exposing those with dementia to these types of environments, Jean explains, allows seniors to recall memories that are considered experiential, not cognitive.

Services are usually brief and carefully planned, with much congregate singing – usually the first stanza of a hymn only. I was fortunate enough to attend a recent service at the First Presbyterian Church in Garden Grove, California. I watched as the participants clamored off their buses, awkwardly pushing walkers and those with verbal capabilities asking questions of or greeting the volunteers. Interestingly, the hubbub ceased as the attendees entered the sanctuary. Several men removed their caps as they were led inside, and throughout the 30-minute service few stirred. With the exception of one woman who rose for a moment, not one person of the 45 seniors in attendance moved or created a disturbance throughout the service. As anyone who works with dementia can attest, this last feat is astounding, since the attention span of those afflicted is usually that of only a few minutes.

The service began with hymn singing, a brief colorful slide presentation of natures' wonders tied in with a short homily and scriptures referring to the majesty of God. The pastor spoke carefully, but not condescendingly and shared simple biblical, life-affirming truths. The service concluded with the recitation of the "Lord's Prayer" (which nearly everyone was able to articulate) and the singing of one last hymn. The group was then escorted to the nearby church hall for a luncheon hosted by the outreach team of volunteers. The atmosphere was welcoming and kind.

Synagogue services have also drawn participant reaction, sometimes to the delight and surprise of the caregiver. "We have seen non-verbal seniors chanting along with the cantor, and one woman was very determined, as is tradition, to touch the Torah and then kiss her fingers" said Jacque Schweppe of the Interfaith Council. "Her daughter could not believe that her mother, who had regressed so much over the last few years, remembered these things. She was very deeply touched by her mother's fierce desire to take part in this worship time." It also reinforced to me the loveliness of the opportunity that was created for mother and daughter to share in such a meaningful experience.

Dementia represents great loss, but like these families you can still find ways in which to create new and loving memories that can mark this period in the journey. The despair that is so easy to dwell on can be put aside when you shift your focus on what can be gained. Remember that despite what is gone, there is still life, and where there is life, there is always hope – hope for peace and even joy! That hope will keep and sustain you and your loved one despite the difficulties of living with dementia. Choose to surround yourself and your parent with people and beliefs and truths that brim over with life and hope, and let them minister to you as you bless your loved one. As you do so, you will be actively making memories that **nothing** can take away.

ABOUT THE AUTHOR

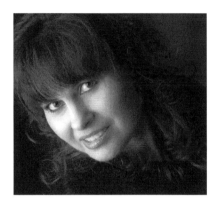 Rosemary De Cuir received her Bachelor of Arts degree in Sociology from California State University, Fullerton in 1986. In 1987 she began her career in the senior services industry as a community relations liaison, marketing director and later as a regional sales and marketing associate for several national assisted living providers. Her experience was augmented by her time serving as supervisor of an Orange County senior center as she sought to expand the day program and foster community support through fundraising, public speaking and writing. She founded Alliance Family Advocates in 2005 and works as a consultant for families, in addition to accepting speaking engagements and training contracts.

Ms. De Cuir was born in Los Angeles and resides in Chino Hills, California.

ISBN 142510118-6

Made in the USA
San Bernardino, CA
21 April 2014